Nursing Research Using Phenomenology

Mary de Chesnay, PhD, RN, PMHCNS-BC, FAAN, is professor at Kennesaw State University, School of Nursing, Georgia. She has received 13 research grants and has authored two books: *Sex Trafficking: A Clinical Guide for Nurses* (Springer Publishing) and the AJN Book of the Year Award winner, *Caring for the Vulnerable: Perspectives in Nursing Theory, Practice and Research*, now in its third edition (with a fourth edition to be published in 2015). Dr. de Chesnay has published over 21 journal articles in *Qualitative Health Research, Journal of Nursing Management, International Journal of Medicine & Law,* and others. A former dean and endowed chair, she reviews for a variety of professional journals. Dr. de Chesnay is a noted expert on qualitative research and a founding member and first vice president of the Southern Nursing Research Society.

Nursing Research Using Phenomenology

Qualitative Designs and Methods in Nursing

Mary de Chesnay, PhD, RN, PMHCNS-BC, FAAN

EDITOR

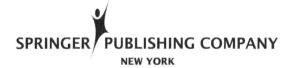

SPRINGER PUBLISHING COMPANY

NEW YORK

Springer Publishing Company, LLC
11 West 42nd Street
New York, NY 10036
www.springerpub.com

Acquisitions Editor: Joseph Morita
Production Editor: Kris Parrish
Composition: Exeter Premedia Services Private Ltd.

ISBN: 978-0-8261-2686-3
e-book ISBN: 978-0-8261-2687-0

Set ISBN: 978-0-8261-7134-4
Set e-book ISBN: 978-0-8261-3015-0

14 15 16 17 / 5 4 3 2 1

The author and the publisher of this Work have made every effort to use sources believed to be reliable to provide information that is accurate and compatible with the standards generally accepted at the time of publication. Because medical science is continually advancing, our knowledge base continues to expand. Therefore, as new information becomes available, changes in procedures become necessary. We recommend that the reader always consult current research and specific institutional policies before performing any clinical procedure. The author and publisher shall not be liable for any special, consequential, or exemplary damages resulting, in whole or in part, from the readers' use of, or reliance on, the information contained in this book. The publisher has no responsibility for the persistence or accuracy of URLs for external or third-party Internet websites referred to in this publication and does not guarantee that any content on such websites is, or will remain, accurate or appropriate.

Library of Congress Cataloging-in-Publication Data
Nursing research using phenomenology : qualitative designs and methods in nursing/ [edited by] Mary de Chesnay.
  p. ; cm.
  Includes bibliographical references.
  ISBN 978-0-8261-2686-3—ISBN 978-0-8261-2687-0 (e-book)
  I. de Chesnay, Mary, editor.
  [DNLM: 1. Nursing Research—methods. 2. Nursing Theory. 3. Qualitative Research.
  4. Research Design. WY 20.5]
  RT81.5
  610.73072—dc23
                                                                        2014028367

Printed in the United States of America by Gasch Printing.

*For Terri Appelhaus, Kathy Donofrio, Laurie Ritchey, and Judy Thon,
and in memory of Phyllis DeLeonardis*

Old friends who are not forgotten . . .
—MdC

CONTENTS

Contributors

Joan L. Bottorff, PhD, RN, FCAHS, FAAN, is professor of nursing at the University of British Columbia, Okanagan campus, faculty of Health and Social Development. She is the director of the Institute for Healthy Living and Chronic Disease Prevention at the University of British Columbia.

Bonnie H. Bowie, PhD, MBA, RN, is associate professor and chair of the Psychosocial and Community Health Nursing Department at Seattle University College of Nursing. She has conducted community-based research and participatory action research on vulnerable populations throughout the Seattle area.

Marlene Z. Cohen, PhD, RN, FAAN, is professor and Kenneth E. Morehead Endowed Chair in Nursing, and the associate dean for research at the University of Nebraska Medical Center, College of Nursing. She has conducted a number of phenomenological studies, mostly focused on persons with cancer, their families, and professional caregivers. She has collaborated with nurses conducting phenomenological research in both the United States and Italy.

Mary de Chesnay, PhD, RN, PMHCNS-BC, FAAN, is professor of nursing at Kennesaw State University and secretary of the Council on Nursing and Anthropology (CONAA) of the Society for Applied Anthropology (SFAA). She has conducted ethnographic fieldwork and participatory action research in Latin America and the Caribbean. She has taught qualitative research at all levels in the United States and abroad in the roles of faculty, head of a department of research, dean, and endowed chair.

Barbara Swore Fletcher, RN, PhD, is assistant professor of nursing at the University of Nebraska Medical Center, College of Nursing. She has conducted several phenomenological studies focused on understanding communication in survivors of head and neck cancer and lymphoma. Her current study uses phenomenological and dyadic quantitative analysis to assess communication between head and neck cancer survivors and their partners. She is currently teaching health promotion and leadership to students in the baccalaureate nursing program.

Rebecca Green, DNS, RN, NCSN, is assistant professor of nursing at Valdosta State University. Her practice background has included neonatal intensive care nursing, pediatric home health nursing, administration and nursing education, clinical trials monitoring, and school nursing. She has conducted qualitative research and published in the areas of vulnerable populations, chronic illness, and innovative pedagogies. She teaches across multiple program levels in diverse content areas such as professional nursing development and community health at Valdosta State University.

Kajsa Landgren, PhD, RN, is a senior lecturer at Lund University, Sweden. Her research focuses on infantile colic. She has studied how infantile colic affects the family and the effect of acupuncture in qualitative and quantitative studies.

Joan Such Lockhart, PhD, RN, CORLN, AOCN, CNE, ANEF, FAAN, is clinical professor of nursing and associate dean for academic affairs at Duquesne University School of Nursing. Dr. Lockhart has conducted phenomenological research focused on the work experience of oncology nurses and nurses' political involvement. She has mentored doctoral students from the United States, Japan, and Lebanon in using phenomenology to explore the health-related experiences of vulnerable populations and caregivers, as well as the work experiences of clinical nurses and nurse faculty.

Tommie Nelms, PhD, RN, is professor of nursing at Kennesaw State University. She is director of the WellStar School of Nursing and coordinator of the Doctor of Nursing Science program. She has a long history of conducting and directing phenomenological research and has been a student of Heideggerian philosophy and research for many years. Her research is mainly focused on practices of mothering, caring, and family.

Lenore K. Resick, PhD, CRNP, FNP-BC, FAANP, is clinical professor of nursing, the Noble J. Dick Endowed Chair in Community Outreach, executive director of the Community-Based Health and Wellness Center for Older Adults, and director of the Family Nurse Practitioner Program at Duquesne University School of Nursing. She has conducted ethnographic and phenomenological research focused on the health of vulnerable populations and advised doctoral students on phenomenological approaches to research.

Donna Sabella, PhD, MEd, MSN, RN, PMHNP-BC, is director of global studies and director of the Office of Human Trafficking, Drexel University's College of Nursing and Health Professions. A mental health nurse, she is interested in hearing people's stories and in qualitative research. She has taught research courses to undergraduate nursing students.

Danuta Wojnar, PhD, RN, MED, FAAN, is associate professor and department chair, Maternal–Child and Family Nursing, Seattle University College of Nursing, Seattle, Washington. She is a Robert Wood Johnson Foundation (cohort of 2012) Executive Nurse Fellow.

FOREWORD

Phenomenology is a descriptive approach to knowledge. It seeks to describe and articulate the fundamental structures—or essences, or grammars—of human experience just as this experience presents itself *to* and *in* and *for* experience. As such, phenomenology can explore the logic of the whole gamut of human experience—from the experience of looking at a work of art to the experience of falling in love with another person, from the experience of perceiving an object in space to the experience of fixing a broken piece of furniture. Any gerund—anything that ends in "-ing"—can be a fruitful field for a phenomenological investigation to be performed to elucidate its structure or grammar as an experience.

Of course, phenomenology's descriptive approach to knowledge can and should also serve a critical function. While phenomenology is not opposed to other ways of knowing, in particular, those ways of engaging and understanding reality practiced in the natural and physical sciences, it does resist the attempt to colonize all knowledge and truth by some practitioners of these empirical sciences. As such, in a field like nursing, phenomenological investigations will offer a critical perspective against natural science approaches that seek to know and affect the human mind and body as physical or material objects open to study only through empirical science and treatable only through physical remedies like medicine or surgery.

A phenomenological approach in the health sciences will ask: What is the essence of the experiences of being diagnosed, being sick, being a patient, being dependent, being hospitalized, recovering, or dying? And, in the nursing field, phenomenology will ask: What is the essence of caregiving, of being present with the dying, of celebrating recovery, and so on?

Phenomenology recognizes that illness, or being ill, for example, is not only a physical phenomenon in an objective sense: Illness is also a lived experience of the subjective, embodied, feeling self. Phenomenology also recognizes that a nurse's work is not only or even primarily scientific work, but human work: The work of a nurse is the work of an embodied subject, a feeling and knowing and experiencing person in relationship to another embodied subject, the patient, who is another feeling and knowing and experiencing person. Phenomenology in nursing is concerned with the subjective, living person in her or his lived body in the experience of health and illness—both nurse and patient. As such, it could have radical effects.

Jeffrey McCurry, PhD
Director, Simon Silverman Phenomenology Center,
Duquesne University, Pittsburgh, Pennsylvania

Series Foreword

In this section, which is published in all volumes of the series, we discuss some key aspects of any qualitative design. This is basic information that might be helpful to novice researchers or those new to the designs and methods described in each chapter. The material is not meant to be rigid and prescribed because qualitative research by its nature is fluid and flexible; the reader should use any ideas that are relevant and discard any ideas that are not relevant to the specific project in mind.

Before beginning a project, it is helpful to commit to publishing it. Of course, it will be publishable because you will use every resource at hand to make sure it is of high quality and contributes to knowledge. Theses and dissertations are meaningless exercises if only the student and committee know what was learned. It is rather heart-breaking to think of all the effort that senior faculty have exerted to complete a degree and yet not to have anyone else benefit by the work. Therefore, some additional resources are included here. Appendix A for each book is a list of journals that publish qualitative research. References to the current nursing qualitative research textbooks are included so that readers may find additional material from sources cited in those chapters.

FOCUS

In qualitative research the focus is emic—what we commonly think of as "from the participant's point of view." The researcher's point of view, called "the etic view," is secondary and does not take precedence over what the participant wants to convey, because in qualitative research, the focus is on the person and his or her story. In contrast, quantitative researchers take pains to learn as much as they can about a topic and focus the research data collection on what they want to know. Cases or subjects that do not provide information about the researcher's agenda are considered outliers and are discarded or treated as aberrant data. Qualitative researchers embrace outliers and actively seek diverse points of view from participants to enrich the data. They sample for diversity within groups and welcome different perceptions even if they seek fairly homogenous samples. For example, in Leenerts and Magilvy's (2000) grounded theory study to examine self-care practices among women, they narrowed the study to low-income, White, HIV-positive women but included both lesbian and heterosexual women.

PROPOSALS

There are many excellent sources in the literature on how to write a research proposal. A couple are cited here (Annersten, 2006; Mareno, 2012; Martin, 2010; Schmelzer, 2006), and examples are found in Appendices B, C, and D. Proposals for any type of research should include basic elements about the purpose, significance, theoretical support, and methods. What is often lacking is a thorough discussion about the rationale. The rationale is needed for the overall design as well as each step in the process. Why qualitative research? Why ethnography and not phenomenology? Why go to a certain setting? Why select the participants through word of mouth? Why use one particular type of software over another to analyze data?

Other common mistakes are not doing justice to significance and failure to provide sufficient theoretical support for the approach. In qualitative research, which tends to be theory generating instead of theory testing, the author still needs to explain why the study is conducted from a particular frame of reference. For example, in some ethnographic work, there are hypotheses that are tested based on the work of prior ethnographers who studied that culture, but there is still a need to generate new theory about current phenomena within that culture from the point of view of the specific informants for the subsequent study.

Significance is underappreciated as an important component of research. Without justifying the importance of the study or the potential impact of the study, there is no case for why the study should be conducted. If a study cannot be justified, why should sponsors fund it? Why should participants agree to participate? Why should the principal investigator bother to conduct it?

COMMONALITIES IN METHODS

Interviewing Basics

One of the best resources for learning how to interview for qualitative research is by Patton (2002), and readers are referred to his book for a detailed guide to interviewing. He describes the process, issues, and challenges in a way that readers can focus their interview in a wide variety of directions that are flexible, yet rigorous. For example, in ethnography, a mix of interview methods is appropriate, ranging from unstructured interviews or informal conversation to highly structured interviews. Unless nurses are conducting mixed-design studies, most of their interviews will be semistructured. Semistructured interviews include a few general questions, but the interviewer is free to allow the interviewee to digress along any lines he or she wishes. It is up to the interviewer to bring the interview back to the focus of the research. This requires skill and sensitivity.

Some general guidelines apply to semistructured interviews:

- Establish rapport.
- Ask open-ended questions. For example, the second question is much more likely to generate a meaningful response than the first in a grounded theory study of coping with cervical cancer.

    Interviewer: Were you afraid when you first heard your diagnosis of cervical cancer?

    Participant: Yes.

    Contrast the above with the following:

    Interviewer: What was your first thought when you heard your diagnosis of cervical cancer?

    Participant: I thought of my young children and how they were going to lose their mother and that they would grow up not knowing how much I loved them.

- Continuously "read" the person's reactions and adapt the approach based on response to questions. For example, in the interview about coping with the diagnosis, the participant began tearing so the interviewer appropriately gave her some time to collect herself. Maintaining silence is one of the most difficult things to learn for researchers who have been classically trained in quantitative methods. In structured interviewing, we are trained to continue despite distractions and to eliminate bias, which may involve eliminating emotion and emotional reactions to what we hear in the interview. Yet the quality of outcomes in qualitative designs may depend on the researcher–participant relationship. It is critical to be authentic and to allow the participant to be authentic.

Ethical Issues

The principles of the Belmont Commission apply to all types of research: respect, justice, beneficence. Perhaps these are even more important when interviewing people about their culture or life experiences. These are highly personal and may be painful for the person to relate, though I have found that there is a cathartic effect to participating in naturalistic research with an empathic interviewer (de Chesnay, 1991, 1993).

Rigor

Readers are referred to the classic paper on rigor in qualitative research (Sandelowski, 1986). Rather than speak of validity and reliability we use other terms, such as accuracy (Do the data represent truth as the participant sees it?) and replicability (Can the reader follow the decision trail to see why the researcher concluded as he or she did?).

DATA ANALYSIS

Analyzing data requires many decisions about how to collect data and whether to use high-tech measures such as qualitative software or old-school measures such as colored index cards. The contributors to this series provide examples of both.

Mixed designs require a balance between the assumptions of quantitative research while conducting that part and qualitative research during that phase. It can be difficult for novice researchers to keep things straight. Researchers are encouraged to learn each paradigm well and to be clear about why they use certain methods for their purposes. Each type of design can stand alone, and one should never think that qualitative research is *less than* quantitative; it is just different.

Mary de Chesnay

REFERENCES

Annersten, M. (2006). How to write a research proposal. *European Diabetes Nursing*, 3(2), 102–105.

de Chesnay, M. (1991, March 13–17). *Catharsis: Outcome of naturalistic research*. Presented to Society for Applied Anthropology, Charleston, SC.

de Chesnay, M. (1993). Workshop with Dr. Patricia Marshall of Symposium on Research Ethics in Fieldwork. Sponsored by Society for Applied Anthropology, Committee on Ethics. Memphis, March 25–29, 1992; San Antonio, Texas, March 11–14, 1993.

Leenerts, M. H., & Magilvy, K. (2000). Investing in self-care: A midrange theory of self-care grounded in the lived experience of low-income HIV-positive white women. *Advances in Nursing Science*, 22(3), 58–75.

Mareno, N. (2012). Sample qualitative research proposal: Childhood obesity in Latino families. In M. de Chesnay & B. Anderson (Eds.), *Caring for the vulnerable* (pp. 203–218). Sudbury, MA: Jones and Bartlett.

Martin, C. H. (2010). A 15-step model for writing a research proposal. *British Journal of Midwifery*, 18(12), 791–798.

Patton, M. Q. (2002). *Qualitative research and evaluation methods* (3rd ed.). Thousand Oaks, CA: Sage.

Sandelowski, M. (1986). The problem of rigor in qualitative research. *Advances in Nursing Science*, 4(3), 27–37.

Schmelzer, M. (2006). How to start a research proposal. *Gastroenterology Nursing*, 29(2), 186–188.

PREFACE

Qualitative research has evolved from a slightly disreputable beginning to wide acceptance in nursing research. Approaches that focus on the stories and perceptions of the people, instead of what scientists think the world is about, have been a tradition in anthropology for a long time and have created a body of knowledge that cannot be replicated in the lab. The richness of human experience is what qualitative research is all about. Respect for this tradition was long in coming among the scientific community. Nurses seem to have been in the forefront, though, and though many of my generation (children of the 1950s and 1960s) were classically trained in quantitative techniques, we found something lacking. Perhaps because I am a psychiatric nurse, I have been trained to listen to people tell me their stories, whether the stories are problems that nearly destroy the spirit, or uplifting accounts of how they live within their cultures, or how they cope with terrible traumas and chronic diseases. It seems logical to me that a critical part of developing new knowledge that nurses can use to help patients is to find out first what the patients themselves have to say.

In the fourth volume of this series, the focus is on phenomenology, perhaps the core of qualitative research. Derived from philosophy, phenomenology seems to me to capture the richness of human experience from the person's point of view in ways that no other design does.

Other volumes address ethnography, life history, grounded theory, historical research, participatory action research, and data analysis. The volume on data analysis also includes material on focus groups and case studies, and two types of research that can be used with a variety of designs, including quantitative research and mixed designs. Efforts have been made to recruit contributors from several countries to demonstrate global applicability of qualitative research.

There are many fine textbooks on nursing research that provide an overview of all the methods, but our aim here is to provide specific information to guide graduate students or experienced nurses who are novices in the designs represented in this series in conducting studies from the point of view of our constituents—patients and their families. The studies conducted by contributors provide much practical advice for beginners as well as new ideas for experienced researchers. Some authors take a formal approach, but others speak quite personally in the first person. We hope you catch their enthusiasm and have fun conducting your own studies.

Mary de Chesnay

Acknowledgments

In any publishing venture, there are many people who work together to produce the final version. The contributors kindly share their expertise to offer advice and counsel to novices, and the reviewers ensure the quality of submissions. All of them have come up through the ranks as qualitative researchers and their participation is critical to helping novices learn the process.

No publication is successful without great people who not only know how to do their own jobs but also how to guide authors. At Springer Publishing Company, we are indebted to Margaret Zuccarini for the idea for the series, her ongoing support, and her excellent problem-solving skills. The person who guided the editorial process and was available for numerous questions, which he patiently answered as if he had not heard them a hundred times, was Joseph Morita. Also critical to the project were the people who proofed the work, marketed the series, and transformed it to hard copies, among them Jenna Vaccaro and Kris Parrish.

At Kennesaw State University, Dr. Tommie Nelms, director of the WellStar School of Nursing, was a constant source of emotional and practical support in addition to her chapter contribution to this volume on phenomenology. Her administrative assistant, Mrs. Cynthia Elery, kindly assigned student assistants to complete several chores, which enabled the author to focus on the scholarship. Bradley Garner, Chadwick Brown, and Chino Duke are our student assistants and unsung heroes of the university.

Finally, I am grateful to my cousin, Amy Dagit, whose expertise in proofreading saved many hours for some of the chapters. Any mistakes left are mine alone.

The body is our general medium for having a world.

—Maurice Merleau-Ponty in *Phenomenology of Perception*

CHAPTER ONE

PHENOMENOLOGICAL PHILOSOPHY AND RESEARCH

Tommie Nelms

*P*henomenological research methods are born out of a long tradition of a philosophy that originated in Germany. While often referred to as the phenomenological movement, there were many different varieties of phenomenological philosophy reflecting very little unity. Edmund Husserl (1859–1938) is considered the father of the phenomenological movement, and for him, the unifying feature was the common conviction that it was only by return to the primary sources of direct intuition and to insights into essential structures derived from them that the great traditions of philosophy with their concepts and problems could be put to use (Spiegelberg, 1982, p. 5). Husserl's phenomenology was a response to what he saw as a crisis in science whereby science was crying out for a philosophy that would restore its contact with the deeper concerns of man (Spiegelberg, 1982, p. 75). Husserl's famous saying "to the things themselves" can be seen as the core of all phenomenological research, indicating the notion that describing lived experience is the essence of phenomenology.

The second most notable figure in the German phenomenological movement was Martin Heidegger (1889–1976). Husserl and Heidegger were senior and junior academic colleagues, often teaching at the same university. Heidegger succeeded Husserl as department chair in Freiburg in 1928, and Husserl hoped Heidegger would further the philosophical work Husserl had begun. While he had initially studied his senior colleague's philosophical work, Heidegger's philosophy went in a very different direction from Husserl's, with a focus on human existence rather than pure ego.

Although he was not considered a phenomenologist in the strictest sense, Hans-Georg Gadamer (1900–2002), a student of Heidegger's, produced work that is often used as the philosophical framework for phenomenological research. Gadamer met both Husserl and Heidegger and considered Heidegger the greatest influence on his thinking. While

Heidegger's philosophy is considered hermeneutic or interpretive phenomenology, Gadamer's philosophy is considered philosophical hermeneutics.
Gadamer focused on the notion of prejudice or prejudgment and its positive,
rather than negative, impact on understanding. For him, language was far
more than a tool; it was the universal horizon of hermeneutic experience. For
Gadamer, the basic mode of understanding for humans was conversation,
whereby a "fusion of horizons" occurred for the conversational partners.

From Germany, the phenomenological movement moved to France
through the works of Jean-Paul Sartre (1905–1980) and Maurice
Merleau-Ponty (1908–1961). Jean-Paul Sartre became acquainted with the
philosophies of Husserl and Heidegger during a period of study in Berlin.
While unique to him, Sartre's philosophy evolved to one that reflected
features of both Husserl and Heidegger as a result of his attention to both
consciousness and existence. From time to time, however, Sartre charged
both Husserl and Heidegger with what he called "bad faith" within their
philosophical systems. Methodologically, Sartre was more like Husserl,
favoring description over explanation, but because his book *Being and Noth-
ingness* reflected a nod to Heidegger's major work, *Being and Time*, he was
referred to as "the French Heidegger." Sartre never referred to himself or
his philosophy as phenomenological, and because of the themes of futility,
despair, and freedom that appear throughout his work, most consider him
an existential philosopher in addition to a novelist, critic, playwright, editor,
and political figure.

The next philosopher in the French phenomenological movement was
Maurice Merleau-Ponty, a friend (although a strained friendship at times) and
colleague of Sartre's. Merleau-Ponty studied both Husserl and Heidegger at
the Sorbonne, but focused more on the philosophy of Husserl. He considered
Husserl's later writings to be key, as opposed to Sartre, who focused more on
Husserl's early work. The dissent between the two French phenomenologists
was reflected in their famous sayings: Merleau-Ponty's "We are condemned
to meaning" and Sartre's "We are condemned to freedom."

Merleau-Ponty's most famous work was titled *The Primacy of Perception*.
By assigning it primacy, Merleau-Ponty did not mean that perception was
privileged, but rather that perception constituted the ground level for all
knowledge and preceded other levels, such as those of the cultural world and
specifically that of science (Spiegelberg, 1982, p. 560). For him, the primary
task was to see and describe how the world presents itself to perception.
Methodologically, Merleau-Ponty was similar to Husserl, advocating bracketing, reduction, and description rather than explanation. As had Sartre,
Merleau-Ponty included the body and embodiment as part of his philosophical system, something lacking in Husserl and Heidegger.

Philosophers like Paul Ricoeur (1913–2005), Emmanuel Levinas (1906–1995), and Jacques Derrida (1930–2004) have also been associated with the phenomenological movement to greater or lesser degrees, and their works have been used as philosophical frameworks for phenomenological research, though not to the extent of the other philosophers noted.

THE PHENOMENOLOGICAL MOVEMENT

The beginning of the phenomenological movement is somewhat difficult to pinpoint. The word "phenomenology" can be traced back through history from Buddhist philosophers to Immanuel Kant, and although used by other philosophers prior to Husserl, its meaning was different then. It is generally agreed that the movement began in the early 1900s with a group of academic philosophers at the University of Gottingen. Like many such movements, it began as a reaction against sociocultural and political forces that were occurring at the time in Germany. One of the main reasons cited for the birth of phenomenology was the progress of the natural sciences and the attempts to view science and scientific methods as the answer to all questions of the natural world as well as human problems and, ultimately, the only route to truth. There were also issues with the decline of speculative philosophy and efforts to convert philosophy into a branch of psychology, labeled psychologism (Spiegelberg, 1982, pp. 19–20). Husserl and those who followed him were intent on creating and using a rigorous human science in the service of human understanding. Their search was for a methodology that would put human science, *Geisteswissenschaften*, on the same footing as the sciences of nature, the *Naturwissenschaften*.

Pinning down a definition of phenomenology can be difficult and is somewhat dependent on the philosophical tradition from which it comes. The term phenomenology comes from the Greek word *phainomenon*, meaning "appearance." Although phenomenology might commonly be called the doctrine of the "intentional structure of consciousness," various philosophers would interpret that definition differently. According to Spiegelberg (1982), "the first objective of the phenomenological approach is the enlarging and deepening of the range of our immediate experience" (p. 679). Meeting this objective was the intent of Husserl's motto, "to the things themselves" (*Zu den Sachen*), whereby phenomena would be afforded a "fuller and fairer hearing" than traditional empiricism had afforded them. Turning to "unadulterated phenomena" requires the "identification and deliberate elimination of theoretical constructs and symbolisms"—not an easy task and one that takes determined effort. It is difficult "to undo the effects of habitual patterns of thought and return to the pristine innocence of *first seeing*" (p. 680). Although difficult, it has been proposed that emancipation from preconceptions and prejudgments is the most teachable aspect of the phenomenological method.

The positivist, empirical notion favoring simplicity and economy in thought, evidenced by Occam's razor, was dismissed by phenomenologists in favor of "a genuine will to know," which requires a spirit of generosity, reverence for the undertaking, and a lens rather than a hammer. While empirics were restricted to sense data only, phenomenologists questioned what other data could be used, noting that simplification may not hold the best access to a legitimate and full picture of reality (Spiegelberg, 1982).

Given that the two main figures of the phenomenological movement were Husserl and Heidegger and that their versions of phenomenology influenced most others, the following section will highlight the major differences in their philosophies, some of which have been cited in the previous discussion. These differences become important when doing phenomenological research because of the essential expectation that phenomenological researchers declare the philosopher whose work underlies their methods and demonstrate allegiance to that phenomenologist's philosophy. This expectation is clearly the case within nursing research, as nursing scholars have developed depth of knowledge and expertise about the various philosophers and their "brands" of phenomenology. There is also an expectation that original works of the selected philosopher have been read and understood by the researcher, in addition to following descriptions or interpretations by others regarding the philosophy.

Husserl's form of phenomenology is considered descriptive or eidetic and is described as the science of the essence of consciousness or an inquiry into the consciousness of the researcher (Porter, 1998). As an epistemology, the researcher or subject calls attention to how the object or experience appears to the consciousness. Husserl's brand requires the use of *bracketing* in an effort to maintain objectivity. With bracketing, the researcher's preconceptions, attitudes, values, and beliefs are held in abeyance to ensure that they do not prejudice the description of the phenomenon. This process within Husserl's phenomenology is also referred to as phenomenological reduction or epoche. Porter (1998, p. 20) described bracketing as "adoption of a doubtful attitude about conventional understandings of the experience." In the final phenomenological description, however, all data—including the researcher's experience with the phenomenon, preconceptions, and assumptions about the phenomenon as well as new insights and understandings about the phenomenon—are used.

Another concept relative to Husserl's brand of phenomenology is *intentionality*, the essential feature of consciousness, meaning that consciousness is directed *toward* an object. When persons are conscious, they are always conscious *of* something, and for humans, that consciousness is of the world. For Husserl, it was the intentionality of consciousness that connected and constituted the object or phenomenon of interest (Spiegelberg, 1982, p. 99). Husserl's intention was the creation of a systematic analysis of consciousness and its objects (Dreyfus, 1987, p. 254). Another essential feature of Husserl's phenomenology is essences or universals as he called them, which are discussed within Spiegelberg's methodological steps.

Heidegger's phenomenological philosophy is considered ontology in that he originally attempted to outline the structure or "constituents" of a human being. His brand of phenomenology is known as hermeneutic or interpretive, given his notion that human beings interpret or attach meanings to their experiences as humans. If, for Husserl, the "wonder of all wonders" was pure ego and pure consciousness, for Heidegger the "wonder of all wonders" was that there is Being (Spiegelberg, 1982, p. 347). Heidegger's philosophy was a study of Being through an investigation of beings (with much significance given to the size of the "B"s). Heidegger believed that Being was revealed by studying beings. Heidegger, unlike Husserl, believed that bracketing or ridding the mind of preconceptions to approach something in a blank way was impossible. How could one explore Being by suspending belief in it? Heidegger did believe, however, that humans were so close or so immersed in being that it was often difficult for them to see without moving away from it to better explore it. This closeness to being or "everydayness" is often taken for granted by humans, but can be revealed through phenomenological questioning and examination. Heidegger might also question the notion that interpretation of a phenomenon is a step beyond description, as outlined by Spiegelberg's method, given his belief that, as human beings, things come to us already interpreted (Finlay, 2009, p. 11).

As evidenced by the title of his work *Being and Time*, Heidegger believed that Being was inextricably tied to and constituted by Time, of which history was a part. Other constituents of the human being were radical finitude, intersubjectivity, involvement with the world, language, and one's concern for one's Being. Heidegger's brand of phenomenology explores the *meaning* of Being for a being or beings in the world. His word for Being, a being, or beings was *Dasein*, which in German means existence or "being there." Heidegger believed that the search to find the meaning of one's life could cause anxiety or unsettledness, and that there could be two reactions to this anxiety for humans. In one case, humans flee the anxiety and fall into conforming to the behavior of others, thus failing to find the unique meaning of their lives and thereby living inauthentically. In the other case, a person stays with the anxiety while pushing forward into the unique possibilities and projects of his or her life, not expecting any final deep meaning, but rather living with authenticity (Dreyfus, 1987, p. 267). For Heidegger, with authenticity come flexibility, aliveness, and joy.

SPIEGELBERG'S PHENOMENOLOGICAL METHOD

According to Spiegelberg (1982), a more common feature of phenomenology than some others was its method, and though none of the early phenomenologists elaborated a system of rules for their methodological procedures, Spiegelberg formulated a method from their philosophies. His steps are as follows: (a) investigating particular phenomena, (b) investigating general essences, (c) apprehending essential relationships among essences, (d) watching modes of appearing, (e) exploring the constitution of phenomena in consciousness, (f) suspending belief in the existence of the phenomena, and (g) interpreting the meaning of phenomena. He noted that while there was general implicit agreement on the practice of the first three steps, the other steps were used by a smaller group. Each of the steps is elaborated.

1. Investigating Particular Phenomena
Three overlapping operations make up this first step, often called "phenomenological description": the intuitive grasp of the phenomena, their analytic examinations, and their description.

   a. Phenomenological Intuiting: Rather than use the term intuition, which has a somewhat mystical connotation, Spiegelberg used the noun form of the verb intuit, "intuiting," to describe this first step. This phase involves *phenomenological seeing*, described as "opening one's eyes," "keeping them open," "not getting blinded," and "looking and listening." In this step, one begins by attempting *to grasp* the uniqueness of the phenomenon by comparing and contrasting it to related phenomena and examining similarities and differences.
   b. Phenomenological Analyzing: This middle phase is an analysis of the phenomenon itself, rather than the expressions that refer to it. Constituents of the phenomenon are distinguished along with "exploration of their relations to and connections with adjacent phenomena"

(Spiegelberg, 1982, p. 691). This step consists of a "general examination of the structure of the phenomena according to the components and their configuration" (p. 692).

c. Phenomenological Describing: According to Spiegelberg, this phase begins in silence and is born out of perplexity and frustration in the face of the phenomena one is trying to describe. Its ultimate function is to provide "unmistakable guideposts to the phenomena" (p. 694) indicative of the uniqueness and irreducibility of the phenomena. Describing affirms the connections between an individual thing and every other thing that denotes or connotes it. The simplest method of description is through negation; other ways are through metaphor and analogy. All describing, however, is selective at best, given the impossibility of exhausting all possibilities.

2. Investigating General Essences (Eidetic Intuiting)
Apprehending a general essence or eidos is the next step in the phenomenological method. An antecedent or exemplifying particular must precede determination of a general essence. The qualities and characteristics of the particular are intuited, leading to awareness of common elements, affinities, patterns, or essences (Spiegelberg, 1982).

3. Apprehending Essential Relationships
This step includes "the discovery of certain essential relationships or connections pertaining to such essences" (p. 699), of which Spiegelberg notes two: relationships within a single essence and relationships between several essences. In examining relationships with a single essence, the concern is whether the components are or are not essential to it. Husserl proposed "free imaginative variation" to deal with this question. Imagine leaving off certain components entirely or replacing them with others and see what happens to the fundamental structure of the phenomenological essence. Either the essence of the phenomenon will remain the same, not requiring the deleted component, or the structure will be essentially changed, indicating a need for the deleted or replaced component. One is cautioned in this process of essential insight, however, to recognize that apprehending essential relationship involves "more than separating an essence into its component parts" (p. 700).

Examining essential relations between several essences also requires imaginative variation, using the same processes of adding and deleting essences to reveal the degree to which they are related. According to Spiegelberg, "it is always the essential nature of the essences in relation to each other which determines their essential relationships" (p. 701). Apprehending essential relationships within a single essence may be called analytical knowledge, while apprehending relationships among several essences suggests synthetic knowledge. The question becomes whether in the relationship to one another, essences are different from what they are alone.

In determining requirements for apprehending essential relationships of either kind, Spiegelberg notes that the features needed for phenomenological insight are both experience and intuition in the face of imagination; "such insights cannot be obtained by mere thinking or reasoning" (Spiegelberg, 1982, p. 702). Imaginative operations into the unique and particular aspects of a case are required, along with efforts to avoid hasty generalization.

4. Watching Modes of Appearing

Phenomenology is the systematic exploration of not only *what* appears but also of the *way* things appear, known as "modes of giveness." *Ways* of appearing are often overlooked in favor of *what* appears. Modes of giveness have to do with the degree to which a whole object can be seen, which is most often not the case. Generally what is seen are facets of an object, while the whole object is assumed to exist. At other times the object is not seen with clarity, but rather is seen through a haze or a veil. An example of appearance in this context is the paintings of the Impressionists.

5. Exploring the Constitution of Phenomena in Consciousness

"Constitution" was a key term in Husserl's phenomenology, indicating that the objects of consciousness were "achievements" of constituting acts (p. 706). Constitution consists of exploring the ways in which a phenomenon establishes itself and takes shape in consciousness. At first things are new, maybe strange, confusing or disorienting, but gradually the newness is integrated into familiar patterns of the world. Constitution is normally spontaneous and passive, but there can be active constitution as one reflects and tries to integrate unrelated phenomena. Either way, constitution begins as small perceptions of an elementary kind that enlarge and merge with past perceptual patterns. According to Spiegelberg (1982), this constituting integration is not by chance associations, but rather follows structural "laws."

6. Suspending Belief in Existence

This step is what is commonly called phenomenological reduction and was considered by Husserl "the master key to phenomenology," although for others it was not common ground (Spiegelberg, 1982, p. 708). Even Husserl himself never fully defined or described the step to his own satisfaction.

The original meaning of phenomenological reduction came from Husserl's mathematics background, whereby the reduction was associated with the mathematical operation of bracketing. The idea is that one detaches the phenomena from everyday experience or the context of natural living "while preserving their content as fully and as purely as possible." One is to suspend judgment "as to the existence or nonexistence of this content" (p. 709).

This step is seen to facilitate genuine intuiting, analyzing, and describing, as it frees one from the usual preoccupation with reality. The reduction should help one to do justice to all data, "real or unreal or doubtful," giving them all equal attention. According to Spiegelberg, phenomenological reduction, which some might view as suspension of the question of existence, does not prevent one from concerns about human existence and its relationship to human essence. As he said, "there is no escape from the earnestness and persistence of the question of reality and of being" (p. 711).

7. Interpreting Concealed Meanings

This last step was most used by hermeneutic phenomenologists. It is seen as a step beyond descriptive phenomenology, and its most complete demonstration was in Heidegger's *Being and Time* (*Sein and Zeit*), as later modified by Sartre, Merleau-Ponty, Gadamer, and Ricoeur. Hermeneutics is an attempt to interpret the sense or meaning of phenomena and hermeneutic phenomenology's "goal is the discovery of meanings which are not immediately manifest to our intuiting, analyzing and describing" (Spiegelberg, 1982, p. 712). The interpreter must go beyond what is immediately given to unveil hidden meanings, which are most often concerned with the problems of human existence and the human situation lived in a mysterious cosmos (p. 714).

In summarizing the significance of the phenomenological approach he outlined, Spiegelberg (1982, p. 716) proposed that it could "be found in its deliberateness and its conscious challenge to the reductionism of Occam's." The phenomenological approach is a deliberate attempt to enrich the world of human experience by bringing out neglected aspects of the experience with the deeper motive of "reverence for the phenomena." "One might describe the underlying unity of the phenomenological procedures as the unusually obstinate attempt to look at the phenomena and to remain faithful to them before even thinking about them" (p. 717). For Spiegelberg, it was not so much a specific step that distinguished phenomenology from other methods as much as "the spirit of philosophical reverence as the first and foremost norm of the philosophical enterprise" (p. 717).

OTHER PHENOMENOLOGICAL METHODS

There are other, more current, phenomenological approaches that nurse researchers use in phenomenolgical research. All of them have formalized the philosophy of one or more of the historical phenomenologists into stepwise processes. Colaizzi (1978), Giorgi (1975), and Van Kaam (1966) were psychologists at Duquesne. They developed a psychological phenomenological method with individual deviations that closely followed the philosophy of Husserl and his three interlocking steps of phenomenological reduction, description, and search for essences. The steps of the Duquesne psychologists' methods are somewhat similar, guiding the researcher to (a) read through all participant descriptions a number of times to get a sense of the whole; (b) extract significant statements; (c) formulate meaning units; (d) collapse the meaning units into themes; (e) analyze and synthesize the meanings; and (f) write an integrated, exhaustive description of the fundamental structure of the phenomenon.

Van Manen (1990) advocated a somewhat different kind of phenomenological method mainly from the Heideggerian tradition. His method of exploring lived experience is an interpretive, artistic approach, the foundations of which are writing and language. According to van Manen, "writing is our method" (p. 124); "writing fixes thought on paper" (p. 125). The writing of the text *is* the research; writing teaches us what we know and the way in which we know it. Writing is a process of self-making and self-consciousness and phenomenological researchers often don't know what they know until it is written down. Writing is also the process that affords the ability to "see" (know, feel, understand) phenomena and as such requires the dialectic of writing and rewriting to create depth of meaning.

Van Manen's process begins with participants writing their lived experience or sharing it with the researcher. Researchers might also closely observe participants in an experience or have them maintain diaries, journals, or logs. Participants' experiences might then be compared to those found in literature, poetry, biographies, autobiographies, or other life histories, as well as artistic materials such as paintings, sculptures, music, or films. Other phenomenological literature about the topic can also be consulted for comparison and dialogue. Phenomenological themes or structures of experience are then explicated. As the analysis and synthesis continue, it is writing that brings forth the meanings, the structures, and the understandings of the phenomenon.

Two of the first nurse researchers to explicate a phenomenological method were Diekelmann and Allen (1989). Their hermeneutic method was in the tradition of Heidegger and Gadamer. Diekelmann also taught the method to nurses and nurse researchers who attended the Heideggerian hermeneutic institutes she led for many years at the University of Wisconsin, Madison. Diekelmann's method was unique in that she supported the notion of research teams, whereby researchers would meet regularly to analyze each other's texts and dialogue about interpretive meanings.

The method begins with the researcher or researchers writing an interpretive summary of each research text, whether interview transcripts, stories, journals, or documents, to get an overall understanding of the text. Teams then come together to discuss the similarities and differences regarding their interpretations of the text(s) and come to a consensus about the meanings, always going back to the text(s) to verify meanings. Researchers then identify relational themes, which are those that cut across all texts. Throughout the interpretive process, texts continue to be read and reread. In the next stage, constitutive patterns are identified. Constitutive patterns are those present in all the documents or texts, and get their name from the Heideggerian ontology in which Heidegger outlined all the characteristics of the human being that made the human being what it was or that "constituted" the human being, such as death, time, world, and other humans. The last stage is preparation of the final interpretive report, using sufficient numbers of excerpts from the texts to support interpretative findings. Rigor in Diekelmann's method was addressed by the use of group consensus or consensual validation. Multiple stages of interpretation also provided a means of bias control (Diekelmann & Allen, 1989).

Another nurse who has developed and disseminated a great deal of expertise regarding phenomenological research methodology is Patricia Munhall (1994, 2012). Munhall entreats researchers "to think phenomenologically" and "be phenomenological" (Munhall, 2012). Although she has explicated a method, she is less concerned with researchers following a formalized process than with their development of a strong depth of knowledge related to the philosophical tenets of phenomenology and the creation of a phenomenological mind set for approaching phenomenological research. Munhall believes that "becoming phenomenologic," as she calls it, leads one to become a "very understanding person." She espouses a flexible method, similar to that of van Manen. Her method is as follows:

1. Immersion
Munhall (2012, p. 122) considers immersion an essential step in which researchers do in-depth study of the philosophy of phenomenology; as she says, "you read, read, read about it." During this beginning stage, it is essential that researchers become familiar with phenomenological philosophers, methods, and different interpretations of phenomenology.

2. Coming to the Phenomenological Aim of the Inquiry
In this stage, there is articulation of the aim of the study. The researchers present their relationship to the study and describe the context and experience(s) that brought them to the study, as well as their present situated contexts. The researchers "decenter" by explicating their assumptions, biases, intuitions, motives, and beliefs in an attempt to come to "unknow." According to Munhall (2012, p. 139), "the state of being decentered and unknowing is challenging to achieve. Unknowing is an art and calls for a great amount of introspection." In the final phase, the aim of the study is articulated in the form of a phenomenological question, whereby the ultimate aim is greater understanding of what it means to be human.

3. Existential Inquiry, Expressions, and Processing
According to Munhall (2012, p. 144), "this stage requires attentiveness, intuitiveness, constant reflection on decentering, active listening, interviews or conversations clarifying, synthesizing, writing, taking photographs, creating verse, and almost anything that will reflect your participant's and your consciousness and awareness of the experience." This stage is similar to what has been described by others as "dwelling," something Munhall believes is essential. She further explicates phases of this stage:

   a. Listen to self and others: develop heightened attentiveness to self and others.
   b. Reflect on personal experiences and expressions.
   c. Provide experiential descriptive expressions: "the experiencer."
   d. Provide experiential descriptive expressions: "others engaged in the experience."
   e. Provide experiential descriptive expressions: the arts and literature.
   f. Provide anecdotal descriptive expressions as experience appears.
   g. Record ongoing reflection in your personal journal.

4. Phenomenological Contextual Processing
According to Munhall, this step parallels the previous step and occurs concurrently with it. In this step the researchers present their thoughts about the

material gathered in step III; the researchers write for the reader, describing situated contexts of those who took part in the study. Further phases of this step are:

   a. Analyze emergent situated contexts.
   b. Analyze day-to-day contingencies.
   c. Assess life worlds.

At this point, Munhall recommends the use of the four components of life worlds—spatiality, corporeality, temporality, and relationality—to further the understandings of study participants, including the researcher (Munhall, 2012, pp. 159–161).

5. *Analysis of Interpretive Interaction*

   a. Integrate existential investigation with phenomenological contextual processing (from Step 4).
   b. Describe expression of meanings (thoughts, emotions, feelings, statements, motives, metaphors, examples, behaviors, appearances and concealments, voiced and nonvoiced language).
   c. Interpret expressions of meaning as appearing from the integration mentioned in *a.*

Munhall (2012, p. 164) cautions against lumping participants' experiences into "acontextual, homogeneous" descriptions of "the one." She urges researchers to highlight the variety of individual, contextual participant experiences with rich descriptions.

6. *Writing the Phenomenological Narrative*

   a. Choose a style of writing that will communicate an understanding of the meaning of this particular experience.
   b. Write inclusively of all meanings, not just the "general" but also the "particular."
   c. Write inclusively of language and expressions of meaning with the interpretive interaction of the situated context.
   d. Interpret with participants the meaning of the interaction of the experience with contextual processing.
   e. Narrate a story that gives voice to the actual language and simultaneously interprets meaning from expressions used to describe the experience.

For Munhall (2012, p. 165), similarities and differences should "show" themselves in the narrative; "the differences are what challenge us and make all the difference in meeting the needs of patients. The differences are paramount in our endeavor to understand individuals in their multiple realities, subjective worlds, life worlds, and individual contingencies."

7. *Writing a Narrative With Implications on the Meaning of Your Study*

   a. Summarize the answer to the phenomenological question with breadth and depth.
   b. Indicate how this understanding, obtained from those who have lived the experience, calls for self-reflection and/or system reflection.
   c. Interpret meanings of these reflections in relation to small and large systems with specific content.
   d. Critique this interpretation with implications and recommendations for political, social, cultural, health care, family, and other social systems.

According to Munhall (2012, p. 169), critique is required to make the experience better for the future; "we do this because in the meaning of our study lies an authentic caring about individuals in experience."

In summary, Munhall (2012) notes that what appears to be many linear steps is actually a multifaceted process that occurs simultaneously and can "flow" from phenomenological philosophy to research into human phenomena. She sees phenomenology as "our hope for understanding in this world" (p. 170). Within phenomenology, Munhall sees optimism, wide-awakeness to experience, reverence for differences and the subsequent possibilities, along with its ability to liberate us from preconceptions and emancipate us from presuppositions that no longer work (p. 171).

RIGOR IN PHENOMENOLOGICAL RESEARCH

While the need for criteria to evaluate the rigor and merit of phenomenological research is seen as critical, specific strategies for assuring, adhering to, and verifying rigor in phenomenological research continue to be the subject of debate. As a qualitative research methodology, many phenomenological researchers have used Lincoln and Guba's (1985) trustworthiness criteria, or the parallel criteria as they are often called, because they parallel the validity and reliability criteria of the positivist paradigm. (And even to imply that there are two research paradigms, qualitative and quantitative, is a debatable issue!) The trustworthiness criteria were posed as four questions in pursuit of the determination of whether "the findings of an inquiry were worth paying attention to" (p. 290). The questions and the related strategies are as follows.

1. Truth Value or Credibility

How can one establish confidence in the "truth" of the findings of a particular inquiry for the subjects (respondents) with whom and the context in which the inquiry was carried out? The researcher must demonstrate the truth value or the credibility with which the multiple constructions of reality are represented (Lincoln & Guba, 1985, p. 290). Three somewhat similar strategies to enhance credibility are prolonged engagement, persistent observation, and triangulation. Prolonged engagement is the investment of sufficient time to meet certain purposes, such as establishing the trust of the respondents, learning the "culture," and testing misinformation and distortions from either the research or the respondents (p. 301). Persistent observation adds depth by identifying those characteristics and elements in the situation that are most relevant to the issue under study, ensuring that sufficient observations are made in favor of premature closure (p. 305). Triangulation can be done with different modes of data collection and different investigators, such as would occur with members of a research team.

Another strategy to enhance truth value of qualitative studies is peer debriefing. Peer debriefing is the notion that a researcher's true peer, who is "disinterested" in the study, will question, challenge, and probe the researcher to expose the researcher's biases, meanings, and assumptions in an effort to keep the inquirer and thus the inquiry "honest" (p. 308). Lincoln and Guba (1985) addressed the notion of negative case analysis whereby hypotheses were revised to account for all known cases without exception. This strategy may be incongruent with phenomenological methods such as Munhall's, in which the aim is not to create a common homogeneous description of "the one," but rather to showcase the variety of participant experiences.

One of the most debated strategies associated with credibility is member checking, which is the process of returning to participants to gather their feedback regarding data they shared with the researcher or the interpretations of the researcher regarding the phenomenon investigated. According to Lincoln and Guba (1985), member checking can be both formal and informal and occurs continuously. While some phenomenologists, such as Colaizzi and van Kaam, have advocated the benefits of member checking, others, like Giorgi, see it as inappropriate to the role of participants to cast them in the role of an evaluator instead of that of a describer of "everyday experience" (Beck, 1994).

2. Applicability or Transferability

How can one determine the extent to which the findings of a particular inquiry have applicability in other contexts or with other subjects (respondents)? Generalizability or external validity is not the purview of qualitative research. The degree to which findings are applicable or transferable to another context is dependent upon the researcher providing enough information for readers to make that determination. The strategy of thick description, whereby the widest possible range of information is provided, allows for judgments of transferability by appliers (Lincoln & Guba, 1985).

3. Consistency or Dependability
How can one determine whether the findings of an inquiry would be repeated if the inquiry were replicated with the same (or similar) subjects (respondents) in the same (or similar) context? Just as there is the notion that there can be no validity without reliability, there is also the notion that without credibility there is no dependability. It may therefore be said that the same strategies that determine credibility in qualitative studies also determine dependability. While the quantitative paradigm advocates replication to ensure dependability, that strategy is incongruent with the notion of emergent design in qualitative studies. The one strategy that is strongly advocated in qualitative and phenomenological studies is the inquiry audit or the audit trail, whereby the processes and products of the study are systematically documented to allow for verification by an auditor (Lincoln & Guba, 1985).

4. Neutrality or Confirmability
How can one establish the degree to which the findings of an inquiry are determined by the subjects (respondents) and conditions of the inquiry and not by the biases, motivations, interests, or perspectives of the inquirer? The major strategy for establishing confirmability is, again, the audit trail, of which triangulation and keeping a reflexive journal are a part. An audit trail consists of the following: raw data, data reduction and analysis, data reconstruction and synthesis, and process notes. For a variety of reasons, qualitative researchers are urged to maintain daily journals or reflexive diaries of activities, insights, musings, and methodological decisions.

Such recordings are helpful as part of the audit trail and also serve as opportunities for reminder, catharsis, and happenings related to one's values and interests (Lincoln & Guba, 1985).

In 1989 Guba and Lincoln published the nonparallel or authenticity criteria. Their belief was that the positivist and constructivist paradigms were too different to have parallel criteria for assessing the rigor of studies and thus there was a need for a new set of criteria that were more closely aligned with the aims of the qualitative paradigm. The authenticity criteria are fairness, ontological authenticity, educative authenticity, catalytic authenticity, and tactical authenticity.

Fairness is "the extent to which different constructions and their underlying value structures are solicited and honored within the evaluation process" (Guba & Lincoln, 1989, p. 245). Ontological authenticity is "the extent to which individual respondents' own constructions are improved, matured, expanded, and elaborated" or "improvement in respondents' conscious experiencing of the world" (Guba & Lincoln, 1989, p. 248). To demonstrate the achievement of this criterion, there must be testimony from respondents or notations at different points within the audit trail of their changed consciousness. Educative authenticity is "the extent to which individual respondents' understanding of and appreciation for the construction of others outside their group are enhanced" (Guba & Lincoln, 1989, p. 248). In addition to testimony from respondents or audit trail notations, respondents must have opportunities to learn of the constructions of others. Catalytic authenticity is "the extent to which action is stimulated and facilitated by the evaluation processes" (Guba & Lincoln, 1989, p. 249). Researchers must provide testimony or reports of such actions. Tactical authenticity "refers to the degree to which stakeholders and participants are empowered to act" (Guba & Lincoln, 1989, p. 250). Again, evidence of tactical authenticity must be provided.

Munhall (1994) developed a methodological system to address the rigor and merit of phenomenological studies called One P, Ten Rs. The One P was the Phenomenological Nod, and the Ten Rs were rigor, which consisted of resonance, reasonableness, representativeness, recognizability, raised consciousness, readability, relevance, revelations, and responsibility. Later Munhall added two more Rs, richness and responsiveness.

The Phenomenological Nod occurs when people reading or hearing the phenomenological description nod in agreement. The first nod should come from the participants who shared their experiences, although all may not agree with all parts of the description (Munhall, 1994). Resonance indicates that the written interpretation of meanings resonates with individuals. Reasonableness relates to the degree to which the interpretation seems reasonable. Representativeness is the adequacy of the interpretation to represent the various dimensions of the experience. Recognizability is when persons who have not necessarily had the experience read it and recognize aspects of an experience and become more acutely aware of it. Raised consciousness is when individuals focus on and gain understanding of an experience they had not considered previously. Readability is when the study reads like a conversation and is easily understood. Relevance is the extent to which studies absorb persons, making them more aware of their humanness and that of others. Revelations highlight something previously concealed. Responsibility reflects being true and faithful to participants, along with ethical considerations and sensitivity to conversations.

Richness is shown when a study reveals a full, embodied, multifaceted, multilayered, thoughtful, sensitive, impassioned description of a human experience. Responsiveness is the degree to which both participants and colleagues respond to the study as important, moving, and capable of releasing them from previously held preconceptions (Munhall, 1994).

Margaret Sandelowski (1986), a nursing qualitative research expert, noted that auditability was one of the main strategies for achieving rigor in qualitative studies and explicated ways to achieve it. According to Sandelowski, auditability is achieved by description, explanation, or justification of the following: (a) how the researcher became interested in the study topic; (b) how the researcher views the thing studied; (c) the specific purpose(s) of the study; (d) how participants or pieces of evidence came to be included in the study and how they were approached; (e) the impact the participants, the evidence, and the researcher had on each other; (f) how the data were collected; (g) how long data collection lasted; (h) the nature of the setting(s); (i) how the data were reduced or transformed for analysis, interpretation, and presentation; (j) how various elements of the data were weighted; (k) the inclusiveness and exclusiveness of the categories developed to contain the data; and (l) the specific techniques used to determine truth value and applicability. For Sandelowski, auditability is demonstrated primarily in the research report.

DEBATED ISSUES IN PHENOMENOLOGICAL RESEARCH

It becomes obvious, as one reads, that phenomenological philosophy and thus phenomenological research is full of variability, which one would expect when the clarity humans seek "is surrounded by halos of vagueness and indefiniteness" (Spiegelberg, 1982, p. 714). This section addresses some of the issues that are debated within the field of phenomenology and phenomenological research.

As stated previously, there is a clear expectation that phenomenologists remain true to a philosopher and his/her philosophical ideas when conducting phenomenological research. There is also a strong expectation that the original works of the chosen philosopher have been read and understood in order for the researcher to remain faithful to the philosophical tradition. One strong criticism of phenomenological researchers is the use of philosophical and methodological ideas that have irreconcilable differences (Finlay, 2009), which can be the case when philosophers with conflicting philosophies and thus methodologies are used to frame a study.

One issue debated is the notion of whether phenomenological description should reveal essential and general structures of a phenomenon (those shared by many) or focus instead on individual experience and thus idiographic details. Halling (2008) argues that both should be accepted. He proposes three levels of analysis: (a) particular experience, such as a person's story; (b) themes common to the phenomenon; and (c) probes for the universal and philosophical aspects of being human. Researchers are counseled to move back and forth between experience and abstraction and between experience and reflection at the different levels.

Historically, there has been a debate about the number of participants or observations required to adequately and successfully reveal a phenomenon under study. The question about numbers might best be addressed by building on the issue of whether or not phenomenology is, or should be, idiographic, general and essential, or universal and reflective of human beings. Early on, Lincoln & Guba (1985) noted that while informational redundancy or data saturation were the criterion measure for the number of participants or observations, it was unusual that a dozen or so participants, if properly selected, would not exhaust most available information, and they recommended the processes of purposive sampling and maximum variation sampling. Giorgi (1975) opined that at least three participants were needed to gather enough variation for an essence. According to Sandelowski (1986), however, the sample size could not be predetermined because it was dependent upon the nature of the data and where the data took the researcher. The best answer to the issue of numbers is the determination of the researcher's purpose; are normative or idiographic understandings being sought?

Another issue of debate is the degree of interpretation researchers should afford their phenomenological descriptions. While recognizing that every experience of a thing is something that has already been interpreted, there are distinctions between descriptive phenomenology and interpretive or hermeneutic phenomenology, with descriptive staying very close to what is given and interpretive moving beyond what is given (Finlay, 2009). Finlay suggests that description and interpretation be viewed as a continuum, whereby phenomenological work is considered more or less interpretative. She supports the notion that hard-and-fast boundaries between description and interpretation limit the spirit of phenomenology.

The issue of researcher subjectivity is another with which phenomenologists struggle. To what extent should researchers bring "their own experience to the foreground" and explore "their own embodied subjectivity" as they strive to explore and describe participants' experiences? For some phenomenologists, the process of reduction or bracketing should render the researcher as "noninfluencial and neutral as possible" (Finlay, 2009, p. 12). Others believe that one's own experiences and understandings cannot be put aside, nor should they be. For most, the best path is a critical awareness of the researcher's preconceived biases and presuppositions in an attempt to separate them from participants' descriptions; striving for openness to the other while acknowledging biases. Too much focus on researcher self-reflection may lead to what has been called "navel gazing," giving too much attention to the researcher's perspective and not enough to the participants'. While some degree of self-knowledge for the researcher is inevitable, the ultimate goal is explication of the participant's perspective and the phenomenon in its appearing leading to a researcher–participant cocreation of data (Finlay, 2009).

Following the previous two issues is the notion of whether or not phenomenology is or should be critical. Is phenomenology to be modernist, whereby truths are sought which are fixed and immutable, or is it to be postmodern, where truths are relative, multivocal, and contingent? Munhall was clear that, to the extent phenomenological findings raise critical consciousness and lead humans to question previously held notions of human experience, it should be done. Finlay (2009) proposed that phenomenology was post postmodern and cited others who challenged phenomenologists to deal with new age messiness, uncertainty, and multivocality, along with cultural criticism and enhanced reflection. Phenomenological knowledge should be seen as "contingent, proportional, emergent, and subject to alternative interpretations" (Finlay, 2009, p. 17).

THE INVISIBILTY OF RECRUITMENT AND RAPPORT

Throughout the explication of phenomenological methods, an area that remains somewhat invisible is the notion of recruitment of participants and the development of rapport with them. Most strategies associated with rigor relate to how data and participants are treated *after* data are collected. The assumption is made that phenomenological researchers will find "good" participants who will share their "lived experiences" truthfully and vividly. While any participant who has lived an experience is said to be as good as any other participant to share the experience, participants who can verbalize, record, or write their experiences with ease and comfort are needed. Participants who "want" to share their experiences with the researcher or who are at least "willing" to share their experiences with the researcher are needed. While there are many experiences about which those who *have lived* or *are living* the experience are anxious to talk and welcome the opportunity to "tell their story," there are other experiences that, for various reasons, persons are hesitant to share with others, especially persons from vulnerable or stigmatized populations.

For example, when I was recruiting mothers who had cared for adult sons who had died of AIDS, a small ad in a major city newspaper resulted in 20 calls from women in 2 days. These women, who experienced "referred stigma" (Goffman, 1963), had had limited opportunity to share their experiences with others. They clearly had a "story to tell" and welcomed a chance to share what they experienced with a nurse (and mother) who wanted to hear what they had lived. In a later study with HIV-infected mothers, I found that having the clinic nurse "vouch" for me as a nurse researcher with integrity was extremely helpful in recruiting participants. In another study of families with a family member in the ICU, a colleague and I found that patients' nurses were essential in recruiting participant families.

The truth value and credibility of research findings are dependent upon the depth and breadth of what participants share with the researcher, and phenomenological research participants need to be made to feel that the researcher has no agenda other than hearing and understanding their experience. Participants require active listening and authentic presencing on the part of the researcher. A true sense of caring to understand the experience of the participant will serve to build rapport, along with not prejudging them and accepting their verbal and emotional expressions. It may also be helpful for researchers to briefly share some information about themselves to "break the ice" and get the conversation started. Participants need assurance that there are no right or wrong answers as they share their experiences.

Another issue faced by phenomenological nurse researchers that may not be faced by researchers from other disciplines is the inclination on the part of the researcher to give advice or health teaching about the experience and/or the inclination to ask for nursing practice information about the experience on the part of participants. While some of the long-acknowledged benefits of participating in qualitative studies for participants are catharsis, self-reflection, healing, empowerment, and sense of purpose that comes with sharing their experience (Hutchinson, Wilson, & Wilson, 1994), if more nursing practice knowledge is desired by participants or deemed necessary by the researcher, arrangements can be made with participants to get the information to them separate from the data collection processes. For example, nurses in the ICU where families were interviewed about their critical illness experiences reported to my colleague and me that families that participated said "the interview with a nurse who cared was better than therapy." In another study, where women were interviewed about their experiences of menopause, a nurse colleague promised the women a class on the pros and cons of hormone replacement therapy after the interviews were completed. Regardless of the tangible or intangible benefits, phenomenological research participants should always be made to feel that their time and their willingness to share their experience are of value and that the understandings gained will be used for good.

FINAL THOUGHTS

At its core phenomenology is both an art and a science, "rigor and resonance" (Finlay, 2009, p. 14). According to Finlay, "research is phenomenological when it involves both rich description of the lifeworld or lived experience, and where the researcher has adopted a special, open phenomenological attitude which, at least initially, refrains from importing external frameworks and sets aside judgments about the realness of the phenomenon" (p. 8). She further noted that "any research which does not have at its core the description of 'the things in their appearing' focusing on experience as lived, cannot be considered phenomenological" (p. 9). For van Manen (1990, p. 13), phenomenology was like poetry, aiming for "an incantative, evocative speaking, a primal telling" in "an original singing of the world." For Spiegelberg (1982, p. 717), "what distinguishes phenomenology from other methods is not so much any particular step It develops or adds to them but *the spirit of philosophical reverence* as the first and foremost norm of the philosophical enterprise." Like nursing, phenomenology is a practice, and while it requires use of the right steps, it also requires a deep understanding of its philosophical underpinnings, along with "an authentic caring about individuals in experience" (Munhall, 2012, p. 169).

REFERENCES

Beck, C. (1994). Reliability and validity issues in phenomenological research. *Western Journal of Nursing Research, 16*(3), 254–267.

Colaizzi, P. (1978). Psychological research as the phenomenologist views it. In R. Valle & M. King (Eds.), *Existential-phenomenological alternatives for psychology* (pp. 48–71). New York, NY: Oxford University Press.

Diekelmann, N., & Allen, D. (1989). A hermeneutic analysis of the NLN criteria for the appraisal of baccalaureate programs. In N. Diekelmann, D. Allen, & C. Tanner, (Eds.), *The NLN criteria for appraisal of baccalaureate programs: A critical hermeneutic analysis* (pp. 11–34). New York, NY: National League for Nursing.

Dreyfus, H. (1987). Husserl, Heidegger and modern existentialism. In B. Magee (Ed.), *The great philosophers: An introduction to western philosophy* (pp. 252–277). London, UK: BBC Books.

Finlay, L. (2009). Debating phenomenological research methods. *Phenomenology and Practice, 3*(1), 6–25.

Giorgi, A. (1975). An application of phenomenological method in psychology. In A. Giorgi, C. Fischer, & E. Murray (Eds.), *Duquesne studies in phenomenological psychology: Volume II* (pp. 72–79). Pittsburgh, PA: Duquesne University Press.

Guba, E., & Lincoln, Y., (1989). *Fourth generation evaluation.* Newbury Park, CA: Sage.

Goffman, E. (1963). *Stigma.* New York, NY : Simon and Shuster.

Halling, S. (2008). *Intimacy, transcendence, and psychology: Closeness and openness in everyday life.* New York, NY: Palgrave Macmillan.

Hutchinson, S., Wilson, M., & Wilson, H. (1994). Benefits of participating in research interviews. *Image: Journal of Nursing Scholarship, 26*(2), 161–164.

Lincoln, Y., & Guba, E. (1985). *Naturalistic inquiry.* Beverly Hills, CA: Sage.

Munhall, P. (1994). *Revisioning phenomenology.* New York, NY: National League for Nursing Press.

Munhall, P. (2012). *Nursing research: A qualitative perspective* (5th ed). Sudbury, MA: Jones & Bartlett Learning.

Porter, E. (1998). On "being inspired" by Husserl's phenomenology: Reflections on Omery's exposition of phenomenology as a method of nursing research. *Advances in Nursing Science, 21*(1), 16–28.

Sandelowski, M. (1986). The problem of rigor in qualitative research. *Advances in Nursing Science, 8*(3), 27–37.

Spiegelberg, H. (1982). *The phenomenological movement: A historical introduction* (3rd revised and enlarged ed.). The Hague, The Netherlands: Martinus Nijhoff Publishers.

Van Kaam, A. (1966). *Existential foundations of psychology.* Pittsburgh, PA: Duquesne University Press.

Van Manen, M. (1990). *Researching lived experience.* Albany, NY: The State University of New York.

CHAPTER TWO

NURSING RESEARCH USING PHENOMENOLOGICAL DESIGNS

Mary de Chesnay

Nurse researchers have conducted many studies using phenomenological approaches. Perhaps because of the philosophy of science courses common to doctoral programs or maybe just because nurses are interested in lived experience, they have established a rich tradition of phenomenological studies in nursing. Phenomenological design has the advantage of focusing on a wide array of phenomena that might be social, cultural, psychological, spiritual, or physiological in nature without the difficulties associated with traveling to foreign settings common to ethnography or spending much time in archives and libraries and poring over historical records. While ethnography and historical research have special appeal, phenomenology enables the researcher to understand not only the person's experience but also the meaning of the experience.

A review of the nursing literature from 1974 to 2014 yielded 329 dissertations in which the phenomenological design was used. Of the dissertations, 15 involved nursing faculty as respondents, 55 involved nursing students, 75 involved clinicians, and 105 involved patients or clients. The remaining samples were miscellaneous, but many of these seemed to involve nursing administrators or leaders. A similar distribution was found in journal literature, but some of those were published in Chinese, Spanish, or Portuguese and could not be analyzed. In particular, the Brazilians seem to have published phenomenological studies. These are discussed later in this chapter.

This chapter highlights some of the recent studies categorized according to focus, with special attention to those in which the study samples were patients or the general population, in which case they would be potential patients. Although many studies were conducted with patient populations or the general public, it seems that nurses have reverted to studying themselves and their students in dramatic numbers. Of the 329 dissertations, for example, more than 200 involved study populations that were either nurses or students. Although much good comes of examining ourselves and our practices, and self-examination is to be expected as we are a study population that has easy access to itself, it would be helpful to know more from the point of view of patients or clients in terms of how they handle their lives as related to health and mental health and what sense they make of their lives. One of the dangers of providing health care is that providers practice from the etic point of view and assume too much about what the patient has to endure and what meaning the patient attaches to the experience.

The categories that are be presented, then, are those with nurses, students, or clinicians as study populations, and attention is given to study populations that experienced an illness or life condition that we as nurses should know about. Because not all dissertations are published, and only abstracts were available for this review, they are discussed separately from studies published in the refereed journal literature. A volume of this size does not allow for a systematic review of the literature on phenomenological studies conducted by nurses, but readers are encouraged to read the originals. Summary information is shown in the tables in this chapter.

DISSERTATIONS

Faculty as Participants

Two examples of faculty as participants are presented here. McGowan (2012) studied the influence of the nurse educator role preparation on teaching methods. She interviewed 11 novice teachers from a national sample and conducted semistructured interviews to analyze through the hermeneutic approach. She then categorized the themes into becoming an educator, planning and processing, and implementing effective teaching strategies.

In contrast to using a national sample, Paulson (2009) interviewed seven nursing faculty at one baccalaureate institution who had worked during the transition from a traditional curriculum to a clinical immersion model. The focus was to study the impact of the new curriculum on faculty resources, and how to meet those challenges.

Students as Participants

Herrera (2012) studied six Hispanic nurses to elicit their stories of progressing through an associate degree nursing program with an objective to examine retention. The researcher audiotaped interviews and examined journals and notes by the students. The themes that emerged were: financial challenges, fear of failing, support, and role models.

Interviews with 16 undergraduate students were analyzed by Moss (2007) to elicit perceptions and meanings of spirituality. The researcher was interested in the students' recognition of spiritual needs, and whether they provided for them in caring for their patients. The three overarching themes were: difficulty in articulating perceptions, lack of preparation to recognize and meet spiritual needs, and asking for permission to include spirituality in their care.

Pham (2011) explored the major stressors of male minority nursing students in baccalaureate education by interviewing 10 students. Four patterns were identified under the overarching theme of "being male is more stressful than being a minority student." The themes were: higher expectations perceived, being outnumbered, being treated differently, and being ridiculed. Pham urged reconsidering how we treat male nursing students.

Clinicians as Participants

A number of dissertations have examined the role of nurses in various specialties. Bender (2009) combined ethnographic methods of participant observation and interviews with patients and nurses in one of Canada's largest tuberculosis (TB) programs. The result was an interpretation of the nature of work that is "welcome intrusions" that included three themes: getting in the door, treating TB but more than that, and central control.

Conte (2011) interviewed 11 pediatric oncology nurses from a children's hospital to examine loss and grief. The themes were: connectedness, doing all one can, and healing. They experienced both connectedness to the family and alienation from those who could not understand how they could perform their work. Alienation also related to protecting themselves and their loved ones from the pain and loss they felt. They discussed the ways by which they sought closure to heal themselves.

Crowe (2012) examined medical–surgical nurses' attitudes toward the homeless by interviewing 11 nurses whose clinical experience ranged from 3 years to 40 years. The five themes were: discovering homelessness, finding common ground, piecing it together, a daily struggle, and relationships based on distrust. The attitude transformation they described enabled them to articulate their daily struggles with maintaining positive nonjudgmental attitudes.

Myers (2000) studied 22 registered nurses who had a parish nursing practice and 19 people who facilitate parish nursing. The process was described as authenticating self through holistic theocentric connecting. They saw parish nursing as a way to provide holistic care in ways they had always wanted to provide it, in the form of a "sacred ministry."

Ten psychiatric nurses were interviewed by Pieranunzi (1992) to examine power and powerlessness, particularly with regard to the split between the biophysical and psychosociocultural models. The two constitutive patterns were the quest for an art and the power of knowing. The themes were: power as connectedness in relationships, being tested by fire, and power as having a voice.

Patients or the General Population as Participants

Of the dissertations found, those that focused on specific illnesses or conditions are highlighted in Table 2.1. The studies represent the diversity in degree-granting institutions around the United States. The central theme seems to be the researcher's interest in the lived experience of the condition by the person who lived it rather than interactions with the health care system or what nurses did with the patients, though the studies clearly have relevance to nursing, and most authors stated the relevance. However, the dissertations themselves were not available, so they are referenced here as abstracts in case readers wish to obtain copies for full review.

Bishop (2005) noted that nurses have long recognized that pregnant women are not immune to violence from their partners. Indeed, some men become violent at the threat of losing the woman's attention to the newborn. Bishop interviewed 11 women who had experienced intimate partner violence during the birth process to discover the meaning of birth, labor, and the postpartum period. Four themes were identified: making it through, control issues, if I could tell nurses, and through a feminist lens.

Bohn (2008) documented the experience of male breast cancer. While much attention is given to female breast cancer, men also can have this diagnosis, but the relatively small number of cases make them somewhat invisible. Bohn interviewed six men who had been diagnosed at least a year but not more than 5 years earlier and stated that saturation had been reached. Ten themes emerged and seemed to point to a new understanding of their vulnerability.

Dunn (1989) had volunteered in a domestic violence shelter and became interested in the stories of battered women. Her interviews with nine women were analyzed according to Giorgi's criteria (1997). The predominant theme was "Living in fear," and the stories were full of anecdotes in which the women lived in fear of their lives, for their children, and for the future. Dunn was the first doctoral student I had who had used the phenomenological design. Though I had studied violence and treated victims of violence, I could not finish reading the draft of Dunn's final dissertation without crying.

Table 2.1 *Dissertations Relating to Patients or General Populations as Sample*

Author (Year)	Topic	Notes
Adam (2012)	Becoming diabetic	10 recently diagnosed adults 3 themes: hearing the news, sorting it out, and moving on
Barron (2000)	Cancer	Margaret Newman's framework 22 adults, varying backgrounds, aged 22–89, with advanced forms of cancer Themes: anguish, coping and hope linked, spirituality, and self-awareness transformation
Bishop (2005)	Meaning of labor, birth, postpartum to women who experienced intimate partner violence in the perinatal period	Feminist framework 11 women's stories from 25 pregnancies Themes: making it through, control issues, if I could tell nurses, through a feminist lens
Bohn (2008)	Male breast cancer	6 men diagnosed within 5 years Themes: deal with it and move on, quest for normalcy and humor, vulnerability among others
Christiansen (1995)	Circumcision in immigrant Somali women	12 Somali women Themes: I am forever changed, living with my past, and anticipating my future
Cordova (2011)	Spirituality among Type II diabetics with macrovascular or microvascular complications	25 male veterans Themes: strongly related to spirituality as supportive factor in coping
Cull-Wilby (1992)	Asthma	9 adults Themes: movement from asthma as gasping for breath to asthma as learning to live with it
Dunn (1989)	Fear in battered women	9 women Theme: living in fear as central concept and how fear defined their activities of daily life
Dyess (2008)	Chronic illness in a faith community	Sample not specified Themes: interaction among the persons, the faith community, and the faith nurse

(continued)

Table 2.1 *Dissertations Relating to Patients or General Populations as Sample (continued)*

Author (Year)	Topic	Notes
Green (2012)	African American parents' experiences in their children's health care encounters	18 parents interviewed Themes: precursory parental relevance and we-relationships
Imberg (2008)	U.S. childbirth for Mexican women	8 Mexican women who had given birth in the United States Themes: safety and security
Iwata (2014)	Japanese men during transition to fatherhood	12 Japanese men Themes: transition to fatherhood, feeling the role of husband and father, sharing time with the child
Jacobson (1991)	Stressful life experiences among 9- to 11-year-old children	12 children Themes: 17 categories of experiences that reflected feeling of loss, being hassled, and threats to self
Jett (2011)	U.S. military after combat-related blast exposure	11 veterans aged 21–over 30 Themes: personal pain and suffering and pain and suffering associated with using the health care system
Kristensen (1992)	Childhood loneliness	14 children 8–10 years old Themes: 9 themes about being alone physically and socially, boredom, anger, authenticity and need for one close relationship
Labore (2012)	Sickle-cell disease	12 young adults 21–25 years old Themes: transition to self-management from care by mothers to care in hospitals to self-care
Lauterbach (1992)	Mother's experience of her baby's death	Feminist framework Sample not specified Themes: perinatal loss, pulling back and recovering, loss and narcissism, and finality of death
Plazas and del Pilar (2011)	Chronic illness	No specific information on sample and findings
Resick (2008)	Health among Russian-speaking women in the United States	12 women aged 40–61 who migrated to the United States but spoke English Themes: health as highly valued, building new life, changes and transitions, trusting self, and importance of hope

(continued)

Table 2.1 *Dissertations Relating to Patients or General Populations as Sample (continued)*

Author (Year)	Topic	Notes
Spratling (2012)	Medically fragile adolescents who require respiratory assistance	11 adolescents aged 13–18 Themes: get to know me, allow me to be myself, be there for me, technology helps, I am an independent person
Subasic (2012)	Hypertrophic cardiomyopathy	Sample not specified Themes: living with, genetic testing, impact on the family and social realtionships
Whyte (2010)	Young women who develop lymphedema after treatment for breast cancer	10 women aged 30–50 Themes: never bothered me, unwanted baggage, who knew, self-preservation, and hopeful determination

JOURNAL LITERATURE

Faculty as Participants

This section includes a brief discussion of several studies that represent the populations of interest. Barss (2012) examined nurse educators' clinical experience using the TRUST model for inclusive spiritual care. The TRUST model includes five domains that generate the acronym: traditions, reconciliation, understandings, searching, and teachers. Developed by the author to address spiritual needs, the model was pilot-tested in an undergraduate program with four female Caucasian faculty members who taught in the program and were trained in the model. Interviews were conducted in the roundtable format, analyzed by the author, and then presented in the form of interpretative poems that included quotes by participants. The nature of participants' experiences was named as "unblocking the bridge," referring to the barriers associated with meeting spiritual needs. Though the sample was small and interviews were conducted only in one setting, the author concludes that the model has great utility for the program in which it was implemented.

Another example of phenomenological research on faculty concerns how faculty members help or hinder students. Poorman, Mastorovich, and Webb (2011) interviewed 30 nurse educators from 18 different nursing programs, including 15 baccalaureate, 10 associate degree, and 5 diploma programs in the United States. When helping students, the participants most commonly referred to "attending," which meant spending time with students and talking with them about their experiences. Attending prevents the danger of premature judgments about the student. For example, one student initially thought to be a poor student was actually spending much time caring for her mother with multiple sclerosis, and it was rather amazing that she could do as well as she did. Beyond simple attending is "understanding," which involves listening and hearing. "Attending as expected" referred to faculty going beyond student expectations of faculty. The results indicated that the teaching–learning process goes beyond process and is a true partnership with emphasis on the student.

Students as Participants

Nursing students are a vulnerable population, but health conditions make selected students even more vulnerable. Ridley (2011) studied students with dyslexia at one university. Seven students with a formal diagnosis were interviewed and results analyzed thematically. Four global themes were identified: dyslexia as a defined disability, as a professional issue, living with dyslexia, and support. The results indicate that even though schools have structures in place for dyslexic students, students are uncertain about how and how much to disclose, and not all faculty provide the level of support these students need. As a caring profession, though, we need to understand these students as caregivers, rather than simply in need of care.

Health literacy is an important aspect of providing care, and there is a question about whether students are being prepared to provide health teaching to the extent that they should. Schekel, Emery, and Nosek (2010) interviewed eight undergraduate nursing students to elicit their experiences in providing health literacy. Three themes emerged from the data: respecting languages, learning persistence; helping patients understand, learning to teach; and promoting engagement, learning sensitivity.

"Respecting languages" example:

> Well, in that situation [diabetes] I gave her pamphlets, but she liked it better when I showed her [she was from Germany].

"Helping patients understand" example:

> A patient was on Coumadin, and instead of talking to them personally about it, they [nurses] just gave them a video.

"Promoting engagement" example:

> *He was in the hospital for medical problems . . . he had a lot of abdominal wounds ... [I]t wasn't just about, let's dress these wounds ... she [nurse] was so non-judgmental. Just everything you hear about how caring a nurse should be.*

The results indicate that faculty should probe logs and journals with students about how they came to their understanding of phenomena instead of simply reading their case studies.

Clinicians as Participants

In this section, one study that demonstrates the application of phenomenology to a core concept of nursing, *Caring*, is presented. Table 2.2 provides a brief overview of other studies with clinicians as participants so that readers may go to the original source if interested in those particular studies.

Table 2.2 *Studies Published in Journal Literature with Clinicians as Participants*

Author (Year)	Topic	Notes
Brykczynski (2011)	Working with women who experienced intimate partner violence	10 advanced practice nurses (APNs) Themes: receptivity, promoting safety, relapsing, celebrating success
de Guzman (2009)	Filipino nurses, attitudes toward geriatric care	7 nurses Themes: the yin and yang of geriatric attitudes—categorized as exhausting/complex and rewarding/educational
Foteini, Vouzavali, Papathanassoglou, Karanikola, Koutroubas, Patiraki, and Papdatou (2011)	Nurse–patient relationship in critical care	12 intensive care nurses Themes: core theme—syncytium, meaning the close connection between nurses and patients and their reciprocal interaction
Holm and Severinsson (2011)	Psychiatric–mental health nursing	Previous research samples Themes: reflective way of being and relationships as foundation for change
Hudacek (2008)	Caring practices of nurses	200 nurses from international sample 7 dimensions: caring, compassion, spirituality, community outreach, providing comfort, crisis intervention, and going the extra distance

(continued)

Table 2.2 *Studies Published in Journal Literature with Clinicians as Participants (continued)*

Author (Year)	Topic	Notes
Iranmanesh, Axelsson, Savenstedt, and Haggstrom (2010)	Caring for the dying by Iranian and Swedish nurses	8 nurses in Iran and 8 in Sweden Themes: sharing space, time to be lost, caring is a learning process
Khalil (2009)	Violence among nurses in Cape Town, South Africa	Mixed design 471 nurses in South Africa Themes: 6 levels of violence
Lyneham, Parkinson, and Denholm (2008)	Intuition in emergency nursing	14 ER nurses Themes: knowledge, experience, connection, feeling, syncretism, and trust

Explicating the complex nature of nursing, Hudacek (2008) collected stories about caring in nursing from 200 nurses and analyzed them using Giorgi's (1997) methodology. Participants were recruited from the Sigma Theta Tau international database through a call for participants in a nursing journal. Nurses who responded with an example of one caring practice were from the United States, Slovakia, Tokyo, Tekrit, Argentina, Australia, and Cuba. Seven dimensions of caring were generated.

1. Caring as the core of nursing
   [W]e developed a relationship that enabled us to manage his pain. I provided spiritual support by arranging for pastoral care. I gave him intellectual and psychological support...I provided his wife with information about her husband's condition.

2. Compassion
   She knew she was sick and dying...I realized at that moment this was another gift of nursing—to help people die well.

3. Spirituality
   I was in the Navy and deployed to Guantanamo Bay Cuba to process Cuban and Haitian refugees. Two of my patients had lost their only sons in an attempted refugee boat trip to the United States. I arranged for a special Mass to be held for healing. The Mass was said in Spanish and English. The entire unit attended.

4. Community Outreach
   In Malawi, Africa, we developed village AIDS committees and provided HIV/AIDS information.

5. Providing Comfort

   He wanted no heroic moments—no machines. We must try to hear the voices of our patients above the din of machinery.

6. Crisis Intervention

   [My patient] had redness that extended down his entire lower abdomen…his physician thought he had a staph infection…he had necrotizing fasciitis.

7. Going the Extra Distance

   I found out that Baby E's mother only had 30 cents with her. I said to the staff: Give me your lunch money…I had more than $60 within a few minutes that would help her.

Patients or the General Population as Participants

Krumwiede and Krumwiede (2012) interviewed 10 Caucasian men aged 62 to 70 with prostate cancer to explore their perceptions and experiences. The mean time since diagnosis was 2.4 years, and most had a radical prostatectomy. All but one were married with supportive spouses. The authors identified themes by using Van Manen's (1999) phenomenology of praxis that represented the men's stories: lived space, lived body, lived time, and lived other. Implications for nursing are to encourage the men to take the time to process the diagnosis before making decisions and to support the patient and his family through the process of deciding and treatment.

George and Thomas (2010) interviewed 10 women aged 65 to 85 in their rural homes to elicit stories of living with diabetes and its complications when living in an isolated area where health care is not readily available and self-management is critical. Of the women, eight were African American and two Caucasian, and all had complications and more than one chronic condition in addition to diabetes. Four themes were identified:

Theme 1: "Your body will let you know. If you miss it you'll wind up in a coma."

Theme 2: "I thought I was fine but I wasn't."

Theme 3: "Only way out is to die."

Theme 4: "You just go on."

The authors stress that health care providers need to identify new and innovative strategies that take into the account the contexts in which patients live their lives for populations like these.

Ward (2011) studied the experience of adults with bipolar disorder who also were substance abusers. Twelve participants were interviewed and data analyzed according to Colaizzi's (1978) method. Six themes emerged: life is hard, feeling the effects, trying to escape, being pushed beyond limits, spiritual support, and a negative connotation. The author stressed that nurses need to do more in the way of teaching self-management and screening for suicidal ideation.

Spratling (2012) interviewed 11 medically fragile adolescents who were on some form of assisted breathing such as ventilators or tracheostomies. Participants ranged from 13 to 18 years and were recruited from an outpatient clinic with five males and six females interviewed. There were seven Caucasian, two African American, one Hispanic, and one mixed African American/Caucasian. Themes were: get to know me, allow me to be myself, be there for me, technology helps, and independence. Because there are few studies on this population, the recommendation is for nurses to increase awareness in general in the community and in nursing programs.

A final example is Ray (2009), in which she interviewed 10 participants (6 soldiers, 2 chaplains, 1 medical assistant, and 1 nurse) who had served in the Canadian military as peacekeepers in Somalia, Rwanda, or the former Yugoslavia and who had been treated for post-traumatic stress disorder upon returning. All had been in recovery for at least 2 years. Themes were: centrality of brotherhood, centrality of time and body, and military response as betrayal. They discussed the nature of brotherhood that develops from close and constant contact during deployment, the connectedness and feeling of loss when brothers were killed, how they maintained a sense of humanity and dissociation, and how it feels to experience the same smells and tastes. Implications are presented not only for nursing care of returning veterans but also for military culture.

See Table 2.3 for selected studies published in nursing journal literature with patients or general populations as samples (2000–2014).

Table 2.3 *Selected Studies Published in Nursing Journal Literature with Patients or General Populations as Samples (2000–2014)*

Author (Year)	Topic	Notes
Bond, Draeger, Mandleco, and Donnelly (2003)	Needs of families with members who suffered traumatic brain injury	7 family members were interviewed Themes: need to know; need for consistent information; need for involvement in care; and need to make sense of the experience

(continued)

Table 2.3 *Selected Studies Published in Nursing Journal Literature with Patients or General Populations as Samples (2000–2014) (continued)*

Author (Year)	Topic	Notes
Cheung and Lee (2011)	Children living with atopic eczema	9 mothers of patients Themes: dealing with extra mothering; giving up their life; becoming an expert; living with blame and worry
DiNapoli (2004)	Adolescent girls and tobacco use	14 girls aged 14–18 Themes: age at initiation, emotional need becoming physiological need, and way of life
Eggenberger and Nelms (2007a)	Family experience when adult member is hospitalized	11 families Themes: Lived space, lived relation, lived body, lived time
Garrett (2010)	Reflections on lived space by child sex abuse survivors	8 men Themes: physical description of home, family space, personal space, secret spaces
Gustafsson, Wiklund-Gustin, and Lindstrom (2011)	Women's reconciliation with suffering from grief	8 women aged 30–72 Themes: no unanimous meaning of reconciliation; narratives had progressive form; survival, discovery, and transformation stories; and analysis of deep structure
Hopkins (2004)	Coping strategies for non-healing leg ulcers	5 (4 men, 1 woman, aged 47–78) Themes: biological disruption; coping and adjustment; social implications; therapeutic relationships
Hughes, Gudmunsdottir, and Davies (2007)	Experiences of urban poor living with cancer	14 cancer patients aged 45–69 (6 men, 8 women) Themes: difficult backgrounds; living with, not dying from cancer; struggling with health care systems and providers

(continued)

Table 2.3 *Selected Studies Published in Nursing Journal Literature with Patients or General Populations as Samples (2000–2014) (continued)*

Author (Year)	Topic	Notes
Hughes, Knibb, and Allan (2010)	Laparoscopic surgery for endometrial cancer	14 women in England Themes: Having cancer; transferring responsibility to the surgeon; information and support; independence, normality
Iaquinta and Larrabee (2004)	Patients with rheumatoid arthritis	6 women, aged 43–67 Themes: grieving while growing; persuading self and others of RA's authenticity; cultivating resilience; confronting negative feelings; navigating health care system; masterminding new lifeways
Jaromahum and Fowler (2010)	Eating after esophagectomy	7 (2 women, 5 men, aged 58–80) Themes: gastrointestinal feelings; fear, positive feelings toward eating
Jonsdottir and Jonsdottir (2007)	Women with COPD who relapse to smoking	7 women aged 45–67 Themes: being caught in spider web; circumstances of relapses; shame, the excuses; ambivalence; incomplete attempts to quit
Kongsuwan, Chaipetch, and Matchim (2012)	Thai Buddhist families' perspective of peaceful death in ICU	9 Thai Buddhist families Themes: knowing death is impending; preparing for peaceful state; not suffering; being with family; families not mourning
Kouwenhoven, Kirkevold, Engedal, and Kim (2012)	Depressive symptoms in acute phase after stroke	9 stroke patients Themes: being trapped; losing oneself
Landgren and Hallstrom (2011)	Parents' experience of living with a baby with infantile colic	23 parents (12 mothers, 11 fathers) Themes: living in inferno; missing situation dreamt of; longing for relaxed closeness; surviving

(continued)

Table 2.3 *Selected Studies Published in Nursing Journal Literature with Patients or General Populations as Samples (2000–2014) (continued)*

Author (Year)	Topic	Notes
Liamputtong, Haritavorn, and Kiatying-Zngsulee (2012)	Thai women living with AIDS	26 Thai women Themes: learning about status; feelings about diagnosis; living positively; constraints
Martins (2008)	Homeless and the health care system	15 homeless adults Themes: living without resources; putting off health care till crisis; barriers; underground resources
Moe, Hellzen, and Enmarker (2013)	Receiving help from home nursing care	6 women, 5 men Themes: being ill and dependent; being at mercy of; feeling inferior
Paguirigan (2012)	Compensated kidney donors in Philippines	11 men, 2 women Themes: sacrificing something important; adversity; altruism; autonomy
Resick (2008)	Health among midlife Russian-speaking women	12 women aged 40–61 Themes: health as highly valued; being a stranger and seeking the familiar; grieving, loss, and building a new life; experiencing change; trusting self; hope
Simpson (2003)	Beliefs about diet and traditional Chinese medicine for Hong Kong women with breast cancer	20 women and 1 other family member Themes: beliefs about foods to eat and not to eat; blending Western and Chinese medicine
Thupayagale-Tshweneagae and Seloilwe (2010)	Emotional violence among women in intimate relationships	10 women Themes: sociocultural practices, age, financial standing, ethnicity, payment of lobola (brideswealth); changing name; changing residence; education; reasons for staying

(continued)

Table 2.3 *Selected Studies Published in Nursing Journal Literature with Patients or General Populations as Samples (2000–2014) (continued)*

Author (Year)	Topic	Notes
Westin, Ohrn, and Danielson (2012)	Nursing home residents encounters with relatives and significant persons	12 residents (5 men, 7 women) aged 78–99 Themes: being pleased; being someone; being inconvenient
Zeigler and Nelms (2009)	Adolescents with implantable cardioverter defibrillators	14 adolescents (9 male, 5 female) Themes: essence—almost normal; life interrupted; still the same, except sometimes it's tough; it cuts both ways; unique joule; living life regular

EXAMPLE OF A RESEARCH PROGRAM

A research program is a set of studies conducted over time that center around a theme, theoretical framework, or methodology. Researchers who are said to have a program of research become experts in their areas as they build knowledge about the phenomenon or methodology and, of course, publish their results so that others may learn from them. In reviewing the literature for this series, the author discovered many nurses who have systematically built research programs. One example is presented here. The author of the following studies also has a chapter in this volume. Nelms works alone or with others from a feminist framework to study the phenomenon of caring, and the concept has taken several forms related to nursing, families, and mothering. In the following studies, her co-authors had been her doctoral students.

The first study found involved a sample of five nurses who related stories of caring (Nelms, 1996). She taught a course in which the graduate students wrote stories of caring and five of the stories inspired her to look further by using Heideggerian hermeneutics to interpret the stories. She then gave her interpretations to the storytellers to validate. In her discussion she presents the nurses as embracing themselves as caring individuals and their patients and students as needing care.

Applying the phenomenological method to mothers whose sons had AIDS, Nelms interviewed 14 mothers (13 White and 1 Black) who had been the primary caregivers for their sons who had contracted AIDS. All of the mothers accepted the homosexuality of their sons—to varying degrees—and they facilitated healing in their family relationships related to their sons' sexual orientation (Nelms, 2000; Nelms & Zeigler, 2008).

In looking at mothers who have HIV/AIDS, Nelms (2005) interviewed 16 women, aged 23 to 54 who were African American (2), African (2), Jamaican (1), and Caucasian (9); two were not identified by race. Six women had been diagnosed during pregnancy, but only two had children who were infected with HIV. They had a total of 42 children; eight of the participants were married and eight were not married. The constitutive pattern that emerged from these data was *burden*. The themes of burden were interconnected but were categorized as: living with the diagnosis, whether to tell children the diagnosis, the unknown future for them and their children, and attempts to relieve the burden by seeking support. The following quotes convey the flavor of their experience.

It's tiring, so tiring... I don't have the energy to be a good mother...(Jane)

...he's the only child I will have, and I want to value him and every experience I have with him. (Alicia)

I just became homeless and a junkie out there for a year, I couldn't face my family, I just wanted to die. (Patricia, upon hearing the diagnosis)

The 11 women who had not revealed the diagnosis to their children wanted to prevent the burden of knowing for their children and the stigma that they thought would attach to the burden. They found ways to relieve the burden for themselves through faith and social support from families and others. The nursing implications of the study remind nurses to keep in mind that mothers with HIV are also women who have their own dreams and needs apart from their children.

When studying units of a family, such as mothers, it is helpful to learn specialized techniques of interviewing families. In the study just discussed, Nelms (2005) interviewed only the mothers, but later worked with Eggenberger to refine methods when families, and not simply individuals within the family, are interviewed. In a study of family experiences when a member is critically ill, Eggenberger and Nelms (2007a, 2007b) interviewed 11 families with 41 members in groups of two to seven members. They point out that traditional family research was usually quantitative and did not take into account the system dynamics. In their study, they paid particular attention to seating, establishing rapport, and sharing information about themselves to establish credibility and ethical issues such as reassurance that choice of whether to participate or not would not influence the care of their family member.

In a secondary analysis of 13 women's breastfeeding stories, Grassley and Nelms (2008, 2009) applied Banks-Wallace's (1998) emancipatory functions of storytelling to further analyze the stories. They independently reviewed the stories to come to an agreement on the exemplars. They concluded that the process of telling the stories might have been emancipatory for the women by examining their experiences. This study nicely illustrates the movement toward meaning in phenomenological research.

FOREIGN LANGUAGE STUDIES

Because some interesting work is coming from other countries and not all journals are published in English, it is important to give credit to these nurse researchers. Information in this section of the chapter comes from the English abstracts, as the journal is published in Portuguese. Discussion is limited by not having access to complete information about the study.

Ciuffo, Rodrigues, and Machaod da Cunha (2009) studied the interactions and rationale of nurses who intervene in child sexual abuse cases. They analyzed speech patterns in nurses to elicit their reasoning about how they interacted with the family and other professionals.

The remaining studies involved participants who were patients or members of the general population. In a study of adolescents forced to have abortions by their mothers, the authors described how the participants described their perceptions of the unsafe procedure and their regrets at not having resisted their mothers' wishes (Domingues et al., 2013).

Another team conducted what they termed a case study using a phenomenological perspective. Chubaci, Merighi, and Yasumori (2005) interviewed a Japanese woman who was experiencing cervical uterine cancer in a hospital in Japan to understand her cultural world.

Batista and Luz (2012) studied the experience of amputation among 12 diabetic patients who described restrictions and limitations imposed by the situation: suffering because of dependence on others, loneliness imposed by social isolation, personal limitations, economic conditions, and/or inadequacy of public policies.

SUMMARY

Areas of Commonality

Although there is great variance among study topics, nurse researchers using phenomenology tend to limit the sample size to 5–20 participants depending on the nature of the topic and accessibility of people who meet the criteria. They specify Colaizzi, Van Manen, Heidegger, or Giorgi when presenting their data. They conduct interviews and rarely supplement these with other types of data collection such as journals or home assessments. For some topics, there had been prior research on the topic, but for others, little had been published, particularly about the lived experience of people with the condition. Rarely did the authors suggest how the phenomenological study could be used as a foundation for intervention research, though the dissertations might have done this in the full study.

Areas of Difference

The most striking difference seemed to lie in the philosophical assumptions about the implication for generalizability. Some authors seem to perceive their work as "standalone" and do not state the sample size as a limitation. This approach is consistent with the idea that qualitative research is rich description without the need for generalizing to any outside the study sample. Others do consider the small sample to be a limitation. This is a strange dichotomy because in qualitative research it is the experience of the participants that is the scope of the study.

A wide range of phenomena were explored, but the study populations could generally be categorized as nurses (faculty, students, clinicians) and the general population (whether or not they were patients). While the experience and meaning of the experience of nursing as a discipline are important, it does seem logical that nurses should be doing more phenomenological research to understand better the contexts in which people live their lives, experience their illnesses and injuries, and make sense of it all. If we understand what the patient understands, we can develop interventions that are not only medically sound, but able to be accepted by the patients.

The literature in nursing was reviewed for examples of phenomenological studies conducted by nurses. The variety of participants ranged from nurses studying themselves to students or faculty with a substantial number of studies conducted with the general population or patients.

REFERENCES

Adam, M. T. (2012). *The lived experience of becoming a diabetic: A phenomenological study* (Doctoral dissertation). Retrieved from Proquest/UMI. (Accession Order No. 2012250575)

Banks-Wallace, J. (1998). Emancipatory potential of storytelling in a group. *Image: The Journal of Nursing Scholarship, 30*, 17–22.

Barron, A. (2000). *Life meanings and the experience of cancer: Application of Newman's research method and phenomenological analysis* (Doctoral dissertation). Retrieved from Proquest/UMI. (Accession Order No. 2002062801)

Barss, K. S. (2012). Building bridges: An interpretive phenomenological analysis of nurse educators' clinical experience using the T.R.U.S.T. model for inclusive spiritual care. *International Journal of Nursing Education Scholarship, 9*, 1–17.

Batista, N., & Luz, M. (2012). Experiences of people with diabetes and amputation of members. *Revue Brasilian Enfermera, 65*(2), 244–50.

Bender, A. C. (2009). *The welcome intrusions of TB nurses: An interpretive phenomenological study of relational work in public health nursing* (Doctoral dissertation). Retrieved from Proquest/UMI. (Accession Order No. 2011033021)

Bishop, S. E. (2005). *The meaning of labor, birth, and the immediate postpartum period for women who have experienced intimate partner violence in the perinatal period* (Dissertation). Abstracts International: Section B: The Sciences and Engineering.

Bohn, M. J. (2008). *Assignment of meaning in the male breast cancer experience: A phenomenological study* (Doctoral dissertation). Retrieved from Proquest/UMI. (Accession Order No. 2010311461)

Bond, A. E., Draeger, C., Mandleco, B., & Donnelly, M. (2003). Needs of family members of patients with traumatic brain injury. *Critical Care Nurse, 23*(4), 63–72.

Brykczynski, K. A. (2011). Intimate partner violence: Advanced practice nurses clinical stories of success and challenge. *Journal of the American Academy of Nurse Practitioners, 23*, 143–151.

Cheung, W., & Lee, R. (2011). Children and adolescents living with atopic eczema: An interpretive phenomenological study with Chinese mothers. *Journal of Advanced Nursing, 68*(10), 2247–2255.

Christiansen, C. D. (1995). *The lived experience of circumcision in immigrant Somali women: A Heideggerian hermeneutic analysis* (Doctoral dissertation). Retrieved from Proquest/UMI. (Accession Order No. 1999030698)

Chubaci, R., Merighi, M., & Yasumori, Y. (2005). A Japanese woman going through cervical uterine cancer: A case study with the social phenomenology approach. *Revista da Escola de Enfermagem, 39*(2), 189–194.

Ciuffo, L., Rodrigues, B., & Machado da Cunha, J. (2009). The nurse in sexual abuse child suspicion attention: A phenomenology approach. *Online Brazilian Journal of Nursing, 8*(3). Retrieved from www.objnursing.uff.br/index.php/nursing/article/view/j.1676-4285.2009.2665

Colaizzi, P. F. (1978). Psychological research as the phenomenologist views it. In R. S. Vale & M. King (Eds.), *Existential phenomenological alternatives for psychology* (pp. 48–71). New York, NY: Plenum.

Conte, T. M. (2011). *Pediatric oncology nurses' lived experiences with loss and grief* (Doctoral dissertation). Retrieved from Proquest/UMI. (Accession Order No. 2012154476)

Cordova, C. M. (2011). *The lived experience of spirituality among type 2 diabetic mellitus patients with macrovascular and/or microvascular complications* (Doctoral dissertation). Retrieved from Proquest/UMI. (Accession Order No. 2012105756)

Crowe, L. E. (2012). *Medical-surgical nurses' attitudes toward patients who are homeless: How attitudes develop and transform* (Doctoral dissertation). Retrieved from Proquest/UMI. (Accession Order No. 2012257780)

Cull-Wilby, B. L. (1992). *Living with asthma: A phenomenological search for meaning* (Doctoral dissertation). Retrieved from Proquest/UMI. (Accession Order No. 1997019389)

De Guzman, A. B. (2009). How many sides does a coin have? A phenomenology of Filipino nurses' motivation and attitudes toward geriatric care. *Educational Gerontology, 35*(3), 260–276.

DiNapoli, P. (2004). The lived experiences of adolescent girls' relationships with tobacco. *Issues in Comprehensive Pediatric Nursing, 27*, 19–26.

Domingues, S. R., Merighi, M., de Jesus, M., & de Oliveira, D. (2013). The experience of women with abortion during adolescence as demanded by their mothers. *Revista Latino-Americana de Enfermagem, 21*(4), 899–905.

Dunn, L. (1989). *The lived experience of fear in battered women* (Doctoral dissertation). Retrieved from Proquest/UMI. (Accession Order No. 1991127848)

Dyess, S. M. (2008). *Living in abundance: The experience of living with chronic illness for adults affiliated with a community of faith with access to a faith community nurse* (Doctoral dissertation). Retrieved from Proquest/UMI. (Accession Order No. 2010418775)

Eggenberger, S., & Nelms, T. (2007a). Being family: The family experience when an adult member is hospitalized with a critical illness. *Issues in Clinical Nursing, 16*, 1618–1628.

Eggenberger, S., & Nelms, T. (2007b). Family interviews as a method for family research. *Journal of Advanced Nursing, 58*(3), 282–292.

Foteini, J. D., Vouzavali, E., Papathanassoglou, E., Karanikola, M., Koutroubas, A., Patiraki, E., & Papadatou, D. (2011). "The patient is my space": Hermeneutic investigation of the nurse-patient relationship in critical care. *Nursing in Critical Care, 16*(3), 140–151.

Garrett, L. (2010). A phenomenological exploration of reflections on lived space by child sexual abuse survivors. *Issues in Mental Health Nursing, 31*, 758–762.

George, S. R., & Thomas, S. P. (2010). Lived experience of diabetes among older, rural people. *Journal of Advanced Nursing, 66*(5), 1092–1100.

Giorgi, A. (1997). The theory, practice, and evaluation of the phenomenological method as a qualitative research procedure. *Journal of Phenomenological Psychology, 28*(2), 235–260.

Grassley, J. S., & Nelms, T. (2008). The breastfeeding conversation: A philosophical exploration of support. *Advances in Nursing Science, 31*(4), 55–66.

Grassley, J. S., & Nelms, T. (2009). Tales of resistance and other emancipatory functions of storytelling. *Journal of Advanced Nursing, 65*(11), 2447–2453.

Green, R. (2012). *African American parents' experiences in their children's health care encounters* (Dissertations, Theses and Capstone Projects: Paper 498). Retrieved from http://digitalcommons.kennesaw.edu/cgi/viewcontent.cgi?article=1498& context=etd

Gustafsson, L., Wiklund-Gustin, L., & Lindstrom, U. (2011). The meaning of reconciliation: Women's stories about their experience of reconciliation with suffering from grief. *Scandinavian Journal of Caring Sciences, 25*, 525–532).

Herrera, A. N. (2012). *Educational journeys of Hispanic women in nursing* (Doctoral dissertation). Retrieved from Proquest/UMI. (Accession No. 2013-99091-036)

Holm, A. L., & Severinsson, E. (2011). A hermeneutic approach to the characteristics of mental health nursing practice. *Journal of Psychiatric and Mental Health Nursing, 18*(10), 843–850.

Hopkins, A. (2004). Disrupted lives: Investigating coping strategies for non-healing leg ulcers. *British Journal of Nursing, 13*(9), 556–563.

Hudacek, S. S. (2008). Dimensions of caring: A qualitative analysis of nurses' stories. *Journal of Nursing Education, 47*(3), 124–129.

Hughes, A., Gudmunsdottir, M., & Davies, B. (2007). Everyday struggling to survive: Experiences of the urban poor living with advanced cancer. *Oncology Nursing Forum, 34*(6), 1113–1118.

Hughes, C., Knibb, W., & Allan, H. (2010). Laparascopic surgery for endometrial cancer: A phenomenological study. *Journal of Advanced Nursing, 66*(11), 2500–2509.

Iaquinta, M., & Larrabee, J. (2004). Phenomenological lived experience of patients with rheumatoid arthritis. *Journal of Nursing Care Quality, 19*(3), 280–289.

Imberg, W. C. (2008). *The meaning of U.S. childbirth for Mexican immigrant women* (Unpublished doctoral dissertation). University of Washington, Seattle.

Iranmanesh, S., Axelsson, K., Savenstedt, S., & Haggstrom, T. (2010). Caring for dying and meeting death: Experiences of Iranian and Swedish nurses. *Indian Journal of Palliative Care, 16*(3), 80–96.

Iwata, H. (2014). The experiences of Japanese men during the transition to fatherhood. *Journal of Transcultural Nursing, 25*(2), 159–166.

Jacobson, G. A. (1991). *The meaning of stressful life experiences as described by nine to eleven year old children: A phenomenological study* (Doctoral dissertation). Retrieved from Proquest/UMI. (Accession Order No. 1993166811)

Jaromahum, J., & Fowler, S. (2010). Lived experiences of eating after esophagectomy: A phenomenological study. *Medsurg Nursing, 19*(2), 96–100.

Jett, S. A. (2011). *The post deployment lived experience of U.S. military troops after combat-related blast exposure* (Doctoral dissertation). Retrieved from Proquest/UMI. (Accession Order No. 2012135383)

Jonsdottir, R., & Jonsdottir, H. (2007). The experience of women with advanced chronic obstructive pulmonary disease of repeatedly relapsing to smoking. *Scandinavian Journal of Caring Science, 21*, 297–304.

Khalil, D. (2009). Levels of violence among nurses in Cape Town public hospitals. *Nursing Forum, 44*(3), 207–217.

Kongsuwan, W., Chaipetch, O., & Matchim, Y. (2012). Thai Buddhist families' perspective of a peaceful death in ICUs. *Nursing in Critical Care, 17*(3), 151–159.

Kouwenhoven, S., Kirkevold, M., Engedal, K., & Kim, H. (2012). "Living a life in shades of grey": Experiencing depressive symptoms in the acute phase after stroke. *Journal of Advanced Nursing, 68*(8), 1726–1737.

Kristensen, K. L. (1992). *The experience of childhood loneliness: Unhappily disconnected* (Doctoral dissertation). Retrieved from Proquest/UMI. (Accession Order No. 1994198373)

Krumwiede, K. A., & Krumwiede, N. (2012). The lived experience of men diagnosed with prostate cancer. *Oncology Nursing Forum, 39*(5), E443–E450.

Labore, N. (2012). *Transition to self-management: The lived experience of 21–25 years old with sickle cell disease* (Doctoral dissertation). Retrieved from Proquest/UMI. (Accession Order No. 2012240289)

Landgren, K., & Hallstrom, I. (2011). Parents' experience of living with infantile colic: A phenomenological hermeneutic study. *Scandinavian Journal of Caring Science, 25*, 317–324.

Lauterbach, S. S. (1992). *In another world: A phenomenological perspective and discovery of meaning in mothers' experience of death of a wished-for baby* (Doctoral dissertation). Retrieved from Proquest/UMI. (Accession Order No. 1994198365)

Liamputtong, P., Haritavorn, N., & Kiatying-Angsulee, N. (2012). Living positively: The experiences of Thai women living with HIV/AIDS in Central Thailand. *Qualitative Health Research, 22*(4), 441–451.

Lyneham, J., Parkinson, C., & Denholm, C. (2008). Intuition in emergency nursing: A phenomenological study. *International Journal of Nursing Practice, 14*(2), 101–108.

Martins, D. (2008). Experiences of homeless people in the health care delivery system: A descriptive phenomenological study. *Public Health Nursing, 25*(5), 420–430.

McGowan, A. R. (2012). *The influence of nurse educator role preparation on faculty teaching methods* (Doctoral dissertation). Retrieved from Proquest/UMI. (Accession Order No. 2012240015)

Moe, A., Hellzen, O., & Enmarker, I. (2013). The meaning of receiving help from home nursing care. *Nursing Ethics, 20*(7), 737–747.

Moss, M. M. (2007). *Nursing students' perceptions of clients' spirituality, spiritual needs, and spiritual care in faith communities* (Doctoral dissertation). Retrieved from Proquest/UMI. (Accession Order No. 2009982076)

Myers, M. E. (2000). *Parish nursing: A process of authenticating self through wholistic theocentric interconnecting* (Doctoral dissertation). Retrieved from Proquest/UMI. (Accession Order No. 2002056062)

Nelms, T. (1996). Living a caring presence in nursing: A Heideggerian hermeneutical analysis. *Journal of Advanced Nursing, 24*, 368–374.

Nelms, T. (2000). The practices of mothering in caregiving an adult son with AIDS. *Advances in Nursing Science, 22*(3), 46–57.

Nelms, T. P. (2005). Burden: The phenomenon of mothering with HIV. *Journal of the Association of Nurses in AIDS Care, 16*(4), 3–13.

Nelms, T., & Zeigler, V. (2008). A study to develop a disclosure to children intervention for HIV-infected women. *Journal of the Association of Nurses in AIDS Care, 19*(6), 461–469.

Paguirigan, M. (2012). Sacrificing something important: The lived experience of compensated kidney donors in the Philippines. *Nephrology Nursing Journal, 39*(2), 107–117.

Paulson, C. (2009). *Faculty teaching experiences in innovative nursing curriculum: An interpretive phenomenological study* (Doctoral dissertation). Retrieved from Proquest/UMI. (Accession Order No. 2010550109)

Pham, T. (2011). *Stressors experienced by male minority student nurses while completing a baccalaureate program* (Doctoral dissertation). Retrieved from Proquest/UMI. (Accession Order No. 2012135533)

Pieranunzi, V. R. (1992). *The hermeneutics of power and powerlessness in psychiatric nursing: A Heideggerian phenomenology* (Doctoral dissertation). Retrieved from Proquest/UMI. (Accession Order No. 1995013806)

Plazas, C., & del Pilar, M. (2011). *Understanding the experience of chronic illness in the age of globalization* (Doctoral dissertation). Retrieved from Proquest/UMI. (Accession Order No. 2012105734)

Poorman, S. G., Mastorovich, M. L., & Webb, C. A. (2011). Helping students who struggle academically: Finding the right level of involvement. *Nursing Education Perspectives, 32*(6), 369–374.

Ray, S. L. (2009). The experience of contemporary peacekeepers healing from trauma. *Nursing Inquiry, 16*(1), 53–63.

Resick, L. (2008). The meaning of health among midlife Russian-speaking women. *Journal of Nursing Scholarship, 40*(3), 248–253.

Ridley, C. (2011). The experiences of nursing students with dyslexia. *Art & Science: Nursing Standard, 25*(24), 35–42.

Schekel, M., Emery, N., & Nosek, C. (2010). Addressing health literacy: The experiences of undergraduate nursing students. *Journal of Clinical Nursing, 19*(5–6), 794–802.

Simpson, P. B. (2003). Family beliefs about diet and traditional Chinese medicine for Hong Kong women with breast cancer. *Oncology Nursing Forum, 30*(5), 834–840.

Spratling, R. (2012). The experiences of medically fragile adolescents who require respiratory assistance. *Journal of Advanced Nursing, 68*(12), 2740–2749.

Subasic, K. (2012). *Living with hypertrophic cardiomyopathy* (Doctoral dissertation). Retrieved from Proquest/UMI. (Accession Order No. 2012257913)

Thupayagale-Tshweneagae, G., & Seloilwe, E. (2010). Emotional violence among women in intimate relationships in Botswana. *Issues in Mental Health Nursing, 31*, 39–44.

Van Manen, M. (1999). The pathic nature of inquiry and nursing. In I. Madjar & I. Walton (Eds.), *Nursing and the experience of illness: Phenomenology in practice* (pp. 17–38). London, UK: Routledge.

Ward, T. D. (2011). The lived experience of adults with bipolar disorder and comorbid substance use disorder. *Issues in Mental Health Nursing, 32*(1), 20–27.

Westin, L., Ohrn, I., & Danielson, E. (2012). Residents' experiences of encounters with relatives and significant persons: A hermeneutic study. *Nursing and Health Sciences, 14,* 495–500.

Whyte, E. (2010). *The lived experience of young women who develop lymphedema after treatment for breast cancer* (Doctoral dissertation). Retrieved from Proquest/UMI. (Accession Order No. 2011284313)

Zeigler, V., & Nelms, T. (2009). Almost normal: Experiences of adolescents with implantable cardioverter defibrillators. *Journal for Specialists in Pediatric Nursing, 14*(2), 142–151.

CHAPTER THREE

LESSONS FROM PHENOMENOLOGICAL STUDIES

Marlene Z. Cohen and Barbara Swore Fletcher

We have both (together and separately) conducted a number of phenomenological studies. When you read the brief methods descriptions in journal articles, you know there is more to the story. This chapter relates some of the stories from the methods of two studies we have conducted. Of course, a major part of the fun of every study is that each raises both similar and unique challenges and questions. Examples from two studies illustrate issues that have arisen for us. We write in the first person, and the "survivor" stories are from a study for which Fletcher was the principal investigator (PI), while the "transplant" stories are from a study for which Cohen was the PI.

STUDY EXAMPLES

A small study was conducted with 30 head and neck cancer (HNC) survivors. The PI was Barb Fletcher. For this study, a master's student graduate assistant (GA) and the PI completed recruitment, and the PI completed all of the one-time interviews. This mixed-methods study assessed factors affecting communication in HNC survivors. The PI and two expert qualitative researchers (Cohen and Schumacher) analyzed the data in this phenomenological study (Fletcher, Cohen, Schumacher, & Lydiatt, 2012).

An example of a larger study was research for which Cohen was the PI, and she worked with an interdisciplinary team to study persons who had hematopoietic stem cell transplantation (HSCT). Data were collected longitudinally for 100 days. This research used mixed methods to study symptoms and quality of life, using quantitative measures, and also included phenomenological interviews at five different times. This required a large team to collect the data, statisticians to analyze the quantitative data, and also researchers with expertise in symptoms, quality of life, and of course, phenomenological research (Cohen et al., 2012; Cohen, Jenkins, Holston, & Carlson, 2013).

GETTING STARTED

Research is very much like a journey. Beginning a study requires passion to carry on despite the inevitable difficulties that will arise along the path. The source of this passion could be clinical experience that makes the researcher feel the topic is important, or the opportunity to work with a team of other researchers. You will learn more about a great idea as the process unfolds. It is also important to think strategically about projects so that they fit in with your focus. Focus makes it easier to carry through in research because the projects build on each other and hopefully are consistent with the other work in which you are engaged.

The transplant study began shortly after I moved to Houston. I had a position at the University of Texas Health Science Center School of Nursing and also with the University of Texas M. D. Anderson Cancer Center. One of the most important things to do in a new place is to find research part- ners who share similar interests and with whom you would like to work. I was very fortunate to meet Dr. Charles S. Cleeland early in my time in Houston. He is the McCullough Professor of Cancer Research, Department of Symptom Research, Division of Internal Medicine, the University of Texas M. D. Anderson Cancer Center, and Department Chair, Department of Symptom Research, Division of Internal Medicine, the University of Texas M. D. Anderson Cancer Center, Houston, Texas. He is a senior scientist and a leader in cancer symptom research who has had a distinguished career and made numerous important contributions. Perhaps even more important, he is as generous with collaborators as he is skilled. When we met, I knew I wanted to work with him, so I started by reading all of his papers—not a small task, as he is a prolific scientist! He invited me to join his weekly research team meetings, and I began to learn a great deal about symptoms. My prior research had focused on the experience of cancer and treatment. We had many discussions about what we might do together and began with a pilot study designed to support an R01 application. The pilot unfolded and he and his team helped tremendously in writing, revising, resubmitting the R01, and finally conducting and publishing the research findings. One of the lessons from this was the value in starting with something small to build a relationship and being sure that our work styles were compatible.

One of the early experiences I had was presenting the study at the institutional review board (IRB) meeting. It was the practice of this IRB to have the PI move to the table around which the IRB members sat and present the study. The team members sat behind the PI and were available to answer any questions with which the PI needed help. I still remember the strong feeling of support they gave me just sitting behind me and being available if I needed them. Mutual support among a strong team is an important ingredient in research.

The lessons from this are to find the right partners, start with something small, a pilot study, and also to be patient with the time it will take, starting as soon as possible and thinking about all the details. While the research was fascinating, working with Dr. Cleeland and the team was clearly the most rewarding part of this work.

PARTICIPANT RECRUITMENT

What I did not realize when I started my first qualitative study was how long recruitment can actually take. I recruited HNC survivors from the clinic where they saw the physician for follow-up. Some days, although there were lots of names on the patient list, after screening with my eligibility criteria, no candidates were available. Sometimes, a few candidates were spread out through the morning or afternoon clinic, but after waiting for several hours, the survivors were not interested in the study. Once, I left the clinic to do some other work and came back in ample time to see the survivor, only to be told that the patient had come into the clinic early and had already seen the physician and left.

In addition to the timing difficulties, I also learned to bring the equipment needed to do the interview with me. More than once, the survivor was willing to complete the interview right then but not necessarily at a later date. I have done interviews in quiet clinic rooms and in physician's offices as well as my own interviewing rooms (more about interviewing later).

Another recruitment challenge I encountered was the survivor who says yes to the study and signs the consent form but is unavailable to complete the interview. I made the mistake during the first small study of holding someone's place with a research number after obtaining consent, but that someone never did participate. This caused a minor logistical problem because several research numbers were never used, and I, as the researcher, had to remember that when dealing with the data that were collected.

In the middle of recruitment for this study, I hired a GA to help. I oriented her to the research and to recruiting subjects. During this process, I noticed that she was talking less and was frequently late for recruitment. I was not sure what to do, and I was considering more training or supervision when I realized that I was making her uncomfortable. Instead of more supervision/training, I reinforced that she was ready to recruit and emphasized the positive (while keeping close tabs on her). With the positive feedback, she blossomed and became a great recruiter and help to the study.

Interviewing

I think by far the most fun activity in qualitative research is the interviewing. HNC cancer survivors can be more difficult to interview because of their speech/communication problems. Their special needs require strategies to facilitate speech/communication. In preparing for an interview, I select a quiet private room with good lighting (part of speech is visual; what is seen on the HNC survivor's face can help to increase understanding of his or her speech). I always make sure that I have Kleenex, cough drops or hard candy, water, or coffee available to help with secretions and the symptom of dry mouth, which the majority of HNC survivors experience. Dry mouth can significantly affect the survivor's ability, ease, and interest in talking. HNC survivors often tell me after the interview, "This is the most I've talked since I got sick!" They often comment that the process of interviewing was helpful to them. While not all informants have similar difficulties with speech, many of the lessons here apply to all interviews. Often people need something to drink as they talk, and when emotions are evoked, tissues are always helpful. Quiet and privacy are always important, and in studies both of us have conducted, informants regularly said how helpful the interview was to them.

Once, when interviewing a person who was a survivor, who had had a laryngectomy, in an empty patient room, I chose to sit directly across from him. People with a laryngectomy breathe through a stoma in the neck and cough and expectorate secretions through that stoma. As the interview progressed the survivor coughed strongly and sputum flew from the stoma and landed on the toe of my shoe. We did not stop talking as I got up and went into the adjoining bathroom and removed the sputum. When I came back, I pulled my chair closer and to the side of the survivor and continued the interview.

Another issue I encountered was the participation of caregivers. In my study, caregivers completed a quantitative booklet but were not interviewed. At times, caregivers expected to be included, and several times patients would not do the interview if the caregiver was not included. In these cases,

I introduced the interview by stating that the survivor was to be interviewed but always allowed caregivers to be involved if they wished.

During one such interview, the patient's wife came and was in the interview room but did not participate. She appeared highly anxious, and this may have been the source of her need to be in the room with the survivor. I provided her with some reading material and had her sit at the far end of the conference table while the survivor and I were on the other end. The survivor was a laryngectomee and had an electrolarynx to communicate but chose to use writing instead to communicate. To begin the interview, he wrote, "The surgery has changed my entire life—everything is different: my job, my home, my family. And she is driving me crazy!" After the interview, the survivor and his family were referred back to the physician for social work and psychological services assistance.

On a different day, I asked another survivor a general question about quality of life and got much more than I asked for. I was interviewing a survivor who was a CEO of his company and who appeared to have few lasting effects from his HNC treatment. He had some swelling and darkening of his face from radiation, his speech was 100% intelligible, and his communication seemed normal. I asked what other things he had learned as a result of the process. He spoke quite eloquently about changes in the way he communicated. He said:

> I used to have a loud booming voice, and I could talk over other people, and I often did. I wasn't angry with other people, just loud. I was used to asking for (and getting) the evidence or data that would back up someone's statement or recommendation. Now my voice is low and gravelly, kind of weak, and I can't make myself heard like I used to. Now I let more junior people run the meeting, and I only step in if I'm needed.

He went on to say that this had led to a change in how he viewed himself and what he felt was important. He now felt that it was good to let others try and let them have the experience. When asked for his opinion, everyone got quiet and listened. He said that he was more relaxed and at peace with himself and the world.

Sometimes what you see is not what you get. One HNC survivor was a big man with tattoos, chains, and a biker jacket. He told me the most amazing story of love about his wife. He said:

> We are kind of a loud family. We like to talk, everybody is loud and boisterous; you know, when I was going through this, and I couldn't speak the way I wanted to speak, and I couldn't talk the way I wanted to talk, I wasn't loud

because of my voice. My wife would sit there and whisper to me, "You tired
yet? You want to go to bed? "She adapted to what I was going through. And I
told her that you don't have to whisper because I can't talk; she goes, "I know
but if you can't be loud, then I'm not going to be loud." I mean when I felt
bad, she felt bad, when I felt good, she felt good. So call it what you want, call
it support, call it love. I just know that she was a strong support structure, a
strong support in my life that helped me get through what I had to get through.
(Fletcher, Cohen, Schumacher, & Lydiatt, 2012)

This same man told me that he did not have anything to complain about. He said he would watch the kids in radiation and the way they just took each day for what it was. He said, "Forget about me, just take the kids! I'm not going to complain as long as there are kids going through this!"

Another interview was with a person who had had a laryngectomy and who used American Indian Sign Language to communicate. He brought his book of signs with him to the interview, and I took approximately 10 minutes to familiarize myself with the signs. The interview was intense because of the alternative communication used. During an interview like this, where no speech is available to record on the tape or the speech has decreased intelligibility, I ask the survivors if it would be OK with them for me to repeat what I think they said, both as a comprehension check and to get the information on the tape for transcription. This procedure worked well, and I have never had a survivor refuse.

Approximately one month later, while recruiting for other survivors, the survivor who used sign language motioned me over and tried to communicate something over and over. After looking at his book, I realized that he was saying that he was dying soon. I was very taken aback by this and got into a conversation with him about it. He said that he had a bad heart. I talked to the resident physician about what had occurred and shortly after that, the patient was admitted to the hospital. I visited him in the hospital, and the next time I went to see him, he had been transferred to a nursing home where he died peacefully three days later.

So many personal lessons are learned from each interview and each informant. We have both learned important lessons about life's priorities, end of life issues, and the value of relationships.

RESEARCH STAFF AND "DISTANCE FROM DATA"

One of the problems with a large grant-funded project is the need to hire staff to assist with many of the aspects of the project. This is clearly in the category of a good problem to have! In our transplant study, the staff included three research staff members who collected data with me. These staff members were needed because of the scope of the project. We collected symptom data from 164 patients eight times, quality-of-life data four times, and conducted phenomenological interviews with 60 individuals (20 Latino, 20 African American, and 20 Caucasian) five times. One of our aims was to identify and compare the experiences of African American, Latino, and Caucasian persons having a transplant, including their meaning of quality of life, symptom severity, and prevalence. Therefore, obtaining data from the three ethnic groups that are most often found in Houston was important. One strategy we used was to hire an African American, a Latino, and a Caucasian interviewer to facilitate recruitment and to collect data. The advantage of this was, of course, that far more data could be collected with a team than one researcher could do alone. In addition, the Latino interviewer was fluent in Spanish, so patients who spoke primarily Spanish could be included. The dilemma this posed is that I was then more removed from much of the data, even though I did collect some data. Also, a great deal of attention had to be paid to the quality of the data being collected. Although I was available for questions at any time, I also met weekly with the data collection team. These meetings were spent reviewing any problems that had come up during the previous week in the recruitment activities and the interviews.

These weekly meetings were essential. One week in November, the data collection team members reported that they had recruited no patients that week. In discussing this, I learned that because this was a longitudinal study, the team had realized that patients they recruited in November would have to have data collected during the time they wanted to be off for Christmas. I assured them I would collect data during that time so they could be off and that they should continue to recruit patients.

Although there was a Latino researcher on the team, she did not speak Spanish fluently, and because I also do not speak Spanish, the interviews conducted in Spanish had to be transcribed and then translated before they could be discussed. Although the Latino interviewer heard the feedback weekly about the other interviews, the translation created a time lag, so feedback on these interviews was not as timely as with the other interviews. Reviewing the transcripts was valuable, as conducting phenomenological interviews requires skill that not everyone possesses and, like any skill, improves with practice.

DATA ANALYSIS AND WRITING

The final part of a project is, of course, to publish it. The analysis starts at this point, and it continues through publication of the manuscript because writing and rewriting the manuscript continues during the analytical process. We have both used a variety of processes to analyze data. The process we used in the survivor study was that the two of us met weekly after having each individually analyzed transcripts line by line. At these weekly meetings we discussed the themes and labels. After we had discussed all of the transcripts, the PI prepared a summary of the themes with the text (quotes) that supported each theme. We again reviewed and discussed this and started to write the results section of the manuscript. When we had a draft, the other co-authors reviewed and commented on the themes, and further revisions were made after all of us discussed them.

Creating a timeline and deadlines is important. We presented a poster with the results of this project at the Midwest Nursing Research Society (MNRS) conference. When we returned, we talked about submitting the paper for the MNRS best paper award. These papers were due on June 1, and we started the detailed analysis in April. In retrospect, although we can see this deadline was unrealistic, it helped us move the paper to the top of our priorities. We both knew it was possible that we might not meet the deadline, so it was not discouraging but rather served to help us with the work. The paper was submitted to another journal in August, only a few months later. We discussed sending it to the WJNR journal (the *Western Journal of Nursing Research*) for the best paper award, but waiting nearly a year did not seem like a good option. Setting deadlines, even when not met, can be helpful.

Many lessons are learned from each study. In phenomenological research, it is vital to choose a topic that you feel passionate about and to work with a team with whom you want to share the research journey. Recruitment of participants requires patience because it will likely take longer than you anticipate, which is a lesson learned at each stage of the research process. Interviewing requires creativity and good equipment—a microphone is useful for soft voices. When you are fortunate enough to be able to have a team, perhaps hired by a funded grant, it is vitally important to stay "close" to the team and the data. Collecting some data yourself helps with the analysis and with really understanding the experience. Staying closely in touch with the team is important to prevent learning about problems when it is too late to remedy them. Finally, the fun of data analysis and writing the manuscript is that it is another chance to dialogue with your research team or partner, which helps to clarify the meaning of the experience being studied. While the process nearly always takes longer than expected, it is well worth the time for the enjoyment of the journey.

REFERENCES

Cohen, M. Z., Jenkins, D., Holston, E., & Carlson, E. (2013). Understanding health literacy in patients receiving hematopoietic stem cell transplantation. *Oncology Nursing Forum, 40*(5), 508–515.

Cohen, M. Z., Rozmus, C., Mendoza, T., Padhye, N., Neumann, J., Gning, I., . . . Cleeland, C. (2012). Symptoms and quality of life in diverse patients undergoing hematopoietic stem cell transplantation. *Journal of Pain and Symptom Management, 44*(2), 168–180.

Fletcher, B., Cohen, M. Z., Schumacher, K., & Lydiatt, W. (2012). Blessing and a curse: Head and neck cancer survivors' experiences. *Cancer Nursing: An International Journal for Cancer Care, 35*(2), 126–132.

CHAPTER FOUR

ONCE UPON A TIME: EXPLORING THE LIVED EXPERIENCE OF PROSTITUTION THROUGH NARRATIVE

Donna Sabella

This is my story about how I came to be the honored recipient of the stories of women involved in prostitution, who bravely and generously took themselves back in time, often through times of darkness, despair, and desolation, to share with me what life in the life had been like for them. I am a mental health nurse, drawn to that field partly because of my interest and curiosity about our invisible parts, which, unlike a heart or kidney that is easily identifiable, make us human. I have no stethoscope or thermometer to gauge or measure the patient's essence. Yet what I have is, in more ways, much stronger and more reflective than such tools. It is the patient's story, a story constructed, one beautiful word at a time. I'm in love with words and stories, probably a state of affairs fostered by the linguistic worlds I grew up in. My mother came from the South and each summer when the family ventured there from Philadelphia for a visit, I marveled at the fact that although people there, including that side of my family, spoke English, it was an English I was hard pressed to understand. And back home in Philadelphia, on my father's side of the family, Italian was their first language, and it served to protect my cousins and me, who spoke no Italian, from things kids weren't supposed to hear back in those days. But it also served to create a barrier to communication and understanding at times. Years later, and all grown up, I knew that words were powerful and that while talk could be cheap, talk could also take us places we never imagined and could shed light on things and places that we found dark and hard to reach. Woven together, words could form a tapestry illustrating our life's story as well as help us to make sense of our experiences and of that story. My love of mental health centers grew from hearing that story and using it as much as possible as a means to understand the storyteller from his or her perspective.

Several years ago, while working as a mobile mental health nurse in a large city, a number of clients I was working with, I suspected, were involved in prostitution. While I knew there were numerous programs for their addiction and mental health issues, my search for programs or clinicians who were capable of treating women with a history of prostitution was unsuccessful. I knew that unless the women I was working with could find someone who understood them, their recovery from whatever else was troubling them could be jeopardized. I also wanted to understand as much as possible, and from an emic perspective, what being involved in prostitution was like—with no judgment about any of it. From that personal desire evolved the first steps in connecting with women who would share their stories with me. What began as research at a graduate level for my master's in mental health nursing evolved into a dissertation topic for my doctorate in educational linguistics, for which I took a phenomenological approach to understand the lived experiences of 15 women who had been, but were not at the time of the study, involved in prostitution; these women were from two major American cities. What follows in this chapter is an account of my trials and tribulations of going through the process, as well as actual excerpts from my dissertation and some recommendations and suggestions for the reader.

GETTING STARTED

Many who have been through this process would probably agree with Dickens's (1859) line that it is the best of times and the worst of times. Before I even started writing, there were two issues that fell into the worst of times category for me looming on the horizon: what would my dissertation be about and who would be my chair and on my committee. In my doctoral program we were told to begin thinking about our topic as soon as possible, as through our coursework we could then begin to build toward the dissertation, and come dissertation time, we would be knowledgeable about our chosen area of interest. I had several possibilities in mind and had actually written a 50-page proposal on another topic (exploring the role of embarrassment as an obstacle to speaking for those learning a second language) before my life took me in another direction, and I found myself working with women who had experienced prostitution. Once I settled on the focus of my research, a process that took time and wasn't always easy, as there were so many directions I could head in (so don't be discouraged as you try to find your forest among the trees), I had to find someone who was not just willing to work with me but who appreciated and understood what I wanted to do. My doctoral program was educational linguistics, which focused on a number of things including second language acquisition, sociolinguistics, and narrative. It was not particularly geared toward people's thoughts and feelings, and certainly gave little thought to prostitution. While the faculty were renowned in their respective areas, I was afraid that I would not be able to find a committee, much less one person, willing to work with me, especially because I knew it would require their going into some uncharted territory. I had originally chosen a chair and committee for my first topic, and when I changed direction, my original chair had agreed to stay on out of the kindness of her heart although we both knew this would not be a good fit. After a few frustrating attempts to make that relationship work in a new context, although I adored and respected the faculty member, I realized the wisdom of trying not to fit a square peg in a round hole and began seeking another chair. A word to the wise is not to be afraid to seek out someone who gets it, with whom you feel comfortable, and who is willing to move beyond their own professional comfort level. I was blessed that Kathy said yes. Having a good chair is as crucial as having a good committee.

Another word to the wise is to listen to your chair when she suggests who she thinks would be good on the committee. While you will need to work with them, the chair does as well, and it is important to do your best in making sure everyone selected has a good and respectful working relationship. Your chair probably knows the departmental politics better than you do, so give heed to her suggestions. Because I was intimidated by one of the people Kathy suggested, I would never have invited that faculty member to the table. However, I trusted Kathy's judgment, and he turned out to be very knowledgeable and helpful. In the end, once my topic and committee were in place, I was clearly headed toward the best of times. With those two issues resolved, there was one more hurdle to overcome before I started writing. Prostitution is a controversial topic and semantics had to be considered when speaking and writing about the women. Were they prostitutes, prostituted women, or sex workers? Each term conveyed a different meaning and perspective. Early on, I had to explain what those differences were and how and why I chose to use the terms I did in my dissertation. With that done, I was ready to put pen to paper and get started. What follows are comments about what I did, and why and how I did it, accompanied by excerpts from my actual dissertation where appropriate.

DESCRIPTION OF THE STUDY

I don't believe in busy work. It was important for me to focus on something that I felt I could get the most out of, related to the work I was doing and near and dear to my heart. I knew this would be a major project that would probably wear on me at some point during the process, and I did not want to find myself laboring over something that I felt lukewarm about right from the start. Prior to starting the dissertation, I had been working with women in prostitution and knew that there was a need for clinicians to better understand what the women who had been there had to say about the experience instead of basing their practice on what academics had to say. Because I had been working with this population in my role as a mental health nurse, I was aware of some of what the women had to say but wanted to know more; hence, the focus became the lived experience of prostitution. Below is my actual abstract which offers an overview of the essence of my research (Sabella Monheit, 2010):

Among people most stigmatized and held in contempt worldwide are women involved in prostitution. The women are discounted and discredited by society at large and rarely are they given the opportunity to speak up and talk about themselves and their experiences of being in the life. The present study, through the use of phenomenological and narrative analysis, examines the narratives of 15 women formerly involved in prostitution and takes a narrative phenomenological approach to investigate the lived experience of prostitution and how the women make sense of their experiences in prostitution through narrative. Participants were selected for maximum variation among women formerly involved in prostitution in two large American cities. Personal interviews were conducted with each participant in order to elicit narratives of their experiences; and van Manen's (1990) phenomenological framework was employed to analyze these narratives. This dissertation examines five major themes that emerged from the data: (a) In the Life, (b) The Good, the Bad, and the Ugly, (c) Identity, (d) Agency, and (e) Lived Relation. The findings reveal that prostitution was primarily a means to an end for these women and that, despite many negative aspects of their experiences, a number of positive aspects of being in the life served to keep women involved in prostitution. In addition, the importance of relationships was evident in the women's narratives with regard to their entry, time involved in the life, and exit from prostitution. The women's construction of their identity and experiences in these narratives differed from how the master narratives define and construct their identity and experiences. The findings critically call into question understanding of prostitution derived from master narratives and dominant discourses about this particular population and afford a better understanding of the complex nature of prostitution and the women's diverse experiences. The clinical implications of those findings are discussed in terms of how to work with, support, and provide care and treatment to women involved in prostitution. (pp. vi–vii)

While the preceding extract serves to give an overview of my work, what follows addresses the scholarly significance and implications of my research as described in the dissertation (Sabella Monheit, 2010):

Prostitution has a long and controversial history. During ancient Greek society, it enjoyed social acceptance. Religious leaders such as Augustine and St. Thomas Aquinas condoned it as providing for a need that if left unmet could cause harm worse than the prostitution itself (Jolin, 1994). While outlawed in many places, it is legal in various locations and is frequently viewed as a nuisance crime in places where it is illegal. In spite of its illegality, prostitution is a multibillion dollar industry (Parker, 1998) and exists everywhere, occurring worldwide in small as well as large cities and in both rural and urban areas—and in all likelihood, right in our own backyards. It is all around us.

Furthermore, those involved in prostitution who do seek treatment rely on a number of medical, health care and behavioral services to help address various work-related risks and conditions such as physical violence, infections, sexually transmitted infections (STIs), HIV/AIDS, posttraumatic stress disorder (PTSD), depression, psychosis, suicide attempts, addiction to drugs and alcohol, and unplanned pregnancies (Jeal & Salisbury, 2004; Parker, 1998; Valera, Sawyer, & Schiraldi, 2001; Weiner, 1996; Young, Boyd, & Hubbell, 2000). Health care professionals are involved in treating prostitutes more than they probably realize. Even though they are often considered invisible and often do not seek help of any kind, an overwhelming majority of prostitutes are in need of medical and especially psychological services and as health care professionals it is imperative that we know how to provide competent and integrated services. In their article on using integrative therapy techniques to treat women involved in prostitution, Napoli, Gerdes, and DeSouza-Rowland (2001) state that much more analysis and research on treating women involved in prostitution needs to be done.

In their review of 14 psychology of women textbooks, Farley and Kelly (2000) note that only three mentioned anything at all about prostitution and prostitutes. In the field of mental health, there is a dearth of literature on how to provide care and behavioral treatment to women wishing to exit prostitution. Williamson and Folaron (2001, 2003), for example, talk about the need for nurses in particular to be aware of the specialized needs of prostitutes and the importance of understanding their motivations, risks, protective strategies, and experiences in order to provide meaningful interventions. As an assistant professor of nursing, I also have found very little in the nursing literature and in nursing textbooks which directly speaks of the needs of prostitutes, although screening for domestic violence is common and mandated in health care settings. Even in women's studies programs, little material is available which deals with prostitution among women. Farley and Kelly (2000, p. 30) refer to the "invisibility of prostitution's harm in the health professions," and also point out that when treatment was sought, medical and social service providers were often disrespectful to women in prostitution, a situation verified as well by Zweig, Schlichter, and Burt (2002) who report on how hospital staff have made insensitive remarks to prostitutes being treated for sexual assault, even more than law enforcement officers. Farley (2003a, 2003b) reports that not just the general public but psychotherapists as well view prostitution as banal and deny its harm to the prostitutes altogether. Baker, Case and Polocicchio (2005) address the lack of health information available to sex workers and suggest that health care professionals need to be better educated about the health care needs and experiences of those involved in prostitution.

There is little doubt that there exists a lack of integrated knowledge and information about women involved in prostitution, particularly with regard to how to treat the women. This lack presents an obstacle in treating those involved in prostitution in a knowledgeable, respectful and appropriate manner. One of the major concerns for women wishing to exit prostitution is a lack of sufficient emotional support during the preliminary stages of leaving (Hedin & Mansson, 2003). There is a great need for awareness raising, training, and educating professionals about prostitution (Hester & Westmarland, 2004). The literature documents the lack of knowledge among health care professionals regarding what trafficking and prostitution are about (Williamson & Folaron, 2001) as well as the unprofessional behavior evidenced by some health care providers when they realize they are treating a prostituted or trafficked woman (Hedin & Mansson, 2003). Health care providers and social service professionals undoubtedly have access to and provide treatment to girls and women, some of whom could be prostituted, yet are rarely taught about this vulnerable population in their training, and health care workers need to be educated about the many health problems experienced by this population, particularly with regard to their mental health and counseling needs (Baker et al., 2005; Baker, Wilson, &

Wineberger, 2004; Farley & Kelly, 2000). As previously mentioned, there is a lack of literature in providing therapy to this population, particularly therapy that addresses the woman's involvement in prostitution.

Many of the women I have spoken with and have come into contact with express a similar concern regarding their fear and discomfort in telling their stories to professionals who do not know how to hear their stories. As an honored recipient of stories from women involved in prostitution, I can attest to how horrific, unspeakable, and unimaginable some of their stories are. When the telling requires what Rymes (2001) calls "dangerous listening" on the part of the professional, often the women shut down and end their narrative when they feel the listener is unable to listen and hear. The findings from this study can offer a meaningful contribution regarding how to successfully listen dangerously to the women's stories and to effectively counsel and treat women involved in prostitution. I argue that, unless the prostitution experience is specifically addressed among women in treatment, the silence and harm surrounding that experience will continue to fester within them, hampering healing and successful recovery. Yet to successfully aid the healing, we need to know what needs to be healed. Looking for that information within the women's own stories is an excellent starting point. An often made comment by women involved in prostitution in response to what is said and written about prostitutes and prostitution by those who are not in the life is that nothing should be told "about us without us." Researchers agree that indeed the women argue that they themselves are not being heard and are also being misrepresented (Arrington, 1987; Boynton, 2002; Chancer, 1993; Roberts, 1986). Letting women tell their stories and using what is learned from these narratives regarding how women experience prostitution and being a prostitute as well as how they make sense of their experience in the life can serve to inform treatment and therapists, serve as a tool to transform the self, and serve as a vehicle for recovery. It would be a beginning for them to tell something "about us with us." As previously stated, in the telling, there is healing for the women, and in the listening, there is learning for the therapist. The findings would provide for some of each. (pp. 23–27)

As is true in all research, no study is perfect, nor does a given study capture all aspects of the essence of what is being examined. And that is fine, as we know this to be the case and do not expect perfection. What we do, therefore, is address possible weaknesses or shortcomings in the work in question and offer them up for readers to see. Although I was seeking to understand the true lived experience of a specific phenomenon, I also realized that the

truth was relative to each person sharing her truth. My study did have limitations, and a section was devoted to addressing what they might be (Sabella
Monheit, 2010):

> While the present study revealed a number of interesting and important
> findings, it should be pointed out that there are a number of limitations
> to be kept in mind. The number of participants is limited to 15 women
> who have described their own experiences, thus the findings have
> limited generalizability. In addition, all of the women are no longer
> involved in prostitution and therefore their stories could be different
> from women still involved in prostitution. The women interviewed for
> this research all viewed themselves as prostituted women, a perspective
> that undoubtedly impacts how they see themselves and their world. In
> general, the term *prostituted woman* is used to describe a woman for
> whom prostitution is not something she entered on her own or for the
> sake of being involved in, in and of itself. The term prostituted woman
> implies that the woman got involved because of addiction, a need for
> money with which she has to support herself and perhaps a family, to
> survive on the streets, or because she was tricked or groomed for it by
> boyfriends, pimps or others. Prostitution is not something she actively
> wishes to do and it serves as a means to some other end. In essence,
> prostitution is something that happens to her because of a variety of life
> circumstances. On the other hand, the term sex worker implies that a
> woman has willingly chosen to provide sexual services and doing so is
> not a means but the end itself. Sex workers feel that they do what they
> do because they want to and that they are not victims. I believe there is
> much that can be learned from women in both camps and to that end
> I reached out to women who described themselves as sex workers as
> well. However, my attempts to interview some of those women were
> not successful so one can only wonder how those narratives might have
> compared to the ones collected from the women who did participate.

Other factors to consider include the fact that all of the women had
exited prostitution at the time of the interviews and all but one of the
women in this study had gone through counseling or a recovery or
treatment program of some sort, which possibly has some bearing on
where they are at this point of their lives and how they speak of their
experiences in prostitution. As we will see, a number of them shared
similar phrases in their narratives, which indicates that they could have
been involved in similar treatment contexts. All but two of the women
were involved in street-level prostitution, which again raises the question as to how the narratives and in-the-life experiences of escorts or

legal brothel sex workers, for example, might have compared to those collected here. Another factor to consider is that I was acquainted with seven of the 15 women interviewed, having met them several years prior to the interviews. Of those seven, I maintained casual long distance contact with two of the women as we occasionally met at conferences or through my work and travels. It is very possible that knowing me could have impacted the interview situation, and could have skewed the women's responses and accounts of their experiences.

Goffman (1963, p. 28) speaks of the "wise" person, whom he defines as the person who is not herself stigmatized as is the group in question, and who is seen as normal, but that person "whose special situation has made them intimately privy to the secret life of the stigmatized individual and sympathetic with it, and who find themselves accorded a measure of acceptance, a measure of courtesy membership in the clan." According to Goffman (1963, pp. 27–29), nurses are often considered among the "wise." It is quite possible that because of my work and experience in this area, my role as a nurse, and my acquaintance with a number of the women, I was considered a member of the clan by some of the women. If true, such a perspective about me on their part could have affected the nature and outcome of our interaction. Finally, while there are a number of commonalities and shared experiences noted across the board, it should be noted that no one woman tells another woman's story and that the findings discussed here are not meant to reflect the experiences of all women. The experience of being involved in prostitution or sex work is undoubtedly a unique and complex experience that cannot be captured by one voice or one story.

LITERATURE REVIEW

My dissertation had a rather extensive literature review, as my topic addressed several different areas. As I was looking at a narrative analysis of the stories of women in prostitution and taking a phenomenological perspective, I knew that I would need to provide background about the narrative, prostitution, and phenomenology. Of all the chapters—and I had seven—this required the most planning on my part to ensure that, while I was reviewing literature from different disciplines, everything fit together in a way that made sense and was connected. I began with narrative and reviewed the literature related to narrative and the following: the lived experience and phenomenology; prostitution and public and opposing discourses; identity; therapy; and phenomenology and prostitution. I then provided a literature review related to prostitution and the following: health, mental health, violence, entry, exit, and life experiences. As you can imagine, the chapter is long and runs to over 70 pages, but I believe I did a nice job of making everything fit together as I explained what I was doing and where I would be taking the reader in the first paragraph of Chapter 2: Literature Review (Sabella Monheit, 2010):

> In seeking to understand the life experiences of women involved in prostitution through a phenomenological lens and in seeking to examine the lived experience of the women involved in prostitution via their discourse and narratives, as well as to consider possible treatment implications based on said narratives, this study merges various aspects of personal or autobiographical narrative, prostitution, and behavioral therapy and treatment. Thus, a review of the literature will begin with a general discussion of what narrative is and its use in various disciplines, followed by its relationship to lived experience and phenomenology. Following that I present an overview of the prostitution literature and conclude with a discussion of narrative related to identity and narrative related to therapy. (p. 34)

METHODOLOGY

It was hammered home to me that methodology does not dictate the research questions but that the reverse should be the case: the research questions dictate the methodology. As a mental health nurse, I wanted to understand and know what the women involved in prostitution had to say about their experiences in it. What was it like for them, and how did they make sense of it? I believed that having access to this information would help me to better serve and support the women I was working with at the time. I wanted an emic perspective and was not driven by any particular motivation save to increase my awareness of this phenomenon, which, I expected, would then help me to better help the women. As I noted in the dissertation, the discussion in the literature was largely driven by two opposing points of view: prostitution either victimized a woman or made her a victor. My question was how could I find out if there were other possibilities? And there the word was: phenomenon. To best unlock the experience of this phenomenon, it seemed clear to me that phenomenology was the best key. With that realization I began reviewing the literature and reading up on other studies using phenomenology as well as works and articles by phenomenologists. My job was relatively simple. While there were numerous articles and books about prostitution, most of them came from researchers who had never been directly involved in it. In addition, there was little written by women who had been involved and even less literature that shed light on the lived experience of prostitution. I had found the gap that needed to be filled and that justified the need for my research. The following excerpt argues for the justification of using a phenomenological approach (Sabella Monheit, 2010):

In reviewing the literature, there are a number of things that become obvious. While much has been written about prostitution and its history (Basserman, 1993; Evans, 1979; Ringdal, 2004; Roberts, 1992), there is a lack of research in a number of areas or approaches. Of relevance and interest to this study is the lack of work that takes a phenomenological approach and allows for women to relate their lived experiences in their own words and voices. There is also a noticeable absence of work which takes a narrative approach to the study of prostitution and either collects narratives or utilizes narrative analysis. While there is work and literature which highlights discursive tensions surrounding prostitution, there is little which addresses identity and/or identity tensions. And most noticeable of all is the lack of a body of work that addresses recovery and treatment of women involved in prostitution. While the debate is complex, with positions clearly marked on all sides of the aisle, when it comes to prostitution discourses, it appears that more of the discourse and research appears to be about prostitution and prostitutes than it is of and from prostitutes themselves, regardless of where they stand on the issue, in their own voices telling their own stories. As Scoular (2004, p. 349) states, "there is an absence of prostitute women's voices and experiences" heard within the discussion. Boynton (2002) states that many prostitutes have been excluded from the research, have not had their voices heard, feel that they have been stigmatized by reports of their lives, or feel that they have been misrepresented altogether and have been falsely stereotyped. In her volume, sex worker Oakley (2007, p. 12) states that occasionally an academic will be "thrown our way to spend a year slumming for a story, or someone will publish a memoir, but more frequently, self-representation is a luxury we are denied."

Dalla (2006a) likewise states that not much is known about the women as individuals with unique histories and little is known as well regarding the details of their lives. Of the work done in which prostitutes and sex workers do have a voice, one can distinguish between work done by academics who interview women and use parts of their collected narratives in their discussions, which then appear in various academic journals or scholarly works, and work written and/or compiled by working women and usually sold to mainstream outlets and the popular press. The former tends more to the negative whereas the latter, while it does address the negative, also makes room for the positive aspects of prostitution and being a prostitute or sex worker. Aside from the paucity of literature from the women's perspective wherein they report on their experiences of being involved in prostitution, there is relatively little work that approaches the study of prostitution from a phenomenological perspective. Much of the data collected when researching prostitution is obtained via surveys, structured interviews, or questionnaires. Very little examines the phenomenon from a deeper and wider perspective. In fact, as of this writing, there was only one article found that examined a prostitute's lived experience from a phenomenological approach, which is Tomura's (2009) study of a prostitute's lived experience of stigma. There is also a dearth of research and literature that examines women's narratives in their own right or that takes a narrative approach and uses narrative analysis in examining prostitution and what it means to be a prostitute. Phoenix (1999, 2000) is one of the few researchers who actually refers to the women's stories as narratives and her work examines those narratives to see how the women make sense of prostitution and their being involved in it. However, in spite of her taking a narrative approach, she does not make clear how she analyzes the women's narratives. (pp. 14–16)

Design

Earlier in this text you have been given information about phenomenology, so I will not go over that information again here. However, I would like to offer some information about why I opted for van Manen's (1990) rendition. In reading through the work of several phenomenologists, I found myself most attracted to van Manen's (1990) perspective, as I felt that I understood his approach best and that it afforded me the best opportunity to capture what I was after. Because I was a novice researcher, it was extremely helpful to have him clearly lay out the steps that were involved in this process (see Sabella Monheit, 2010, pp. 155–161) almost as if this were a recipe, and his approach touched upon many of the areas that I felt were important and related to what I wanted to do. I was also very drawn to his inclusion of what he referred to as lifeworld existentials, as these constructs were very much relevant to areas that I wanted to explore. Below is an excerpt from my chapter on methodology and research design that illustrates why I utilized van Manen's framework and what that framework consists of (Sabella Monheit, 2010):

> The present study utilized van Manen's (1990) method of phenome-nology and focused mainly on the content of the narratives, primarily utilizing narrative as the means of obtaining the data. However, some attention was paid to linguistic and grammatical features of the women's narratives and their responses to interview questions, for in the third process of van Manen's (1990) method of phenomenology, detailed below, language, words and linguistic features are indeed objects of exploration. The analysis was mostly thematic in nature and essentially consisted of repeated listening to the audiotaped interviews, and careful, numerous, and thorough readings of the transcripts before as well as during the processes of coding and analyzing the data. The process also involved seeing what categories or themes emerged across the whole dataset as well as from each woman's interview and included coding and selecting data relevant to the study's research question and objectives.
>
> With regard to the RQ, What is the lived experience of prostitution? narrative served as the means by which the experience of what it is like to be involved in prostitution was accessed. The framework here is phe-nomenological in nature as the question seeks to explore the phenom-enon of being a prostitute and being involved in prostitution. As van Manen (1990) states, the goal of phenomenology is to provide us with a deeper understanding of the nature or meaning of our everyday expe-riences. As such, a phenomenological analysis allows the information and themes to emerge from the data on their own. The women were asked to talk about their experiences in prostitution by use of an open-ended prompt with as little interruption or other questions from the researcher as possible and their narratives were taped, transcribed and analyzed in their entirety. The analysis for this question was conducted from a phenomenological perspective and relied on van Manen's (1990) phenomenological method. According to van Manen (1990) as well as others (Groenewald, 2004; Hycner, 1999), researchers using phenome-nology do not like to prescribe techniques as it is felt that one cannot impose a method on a phenomenon. As van Manen (1990, p. 30) states, "the method of phenomenology and hermeneutics is that there is no method" nor is there focus on specific steps in conducting such research. However, van Manen (1990, p. 30) does provide some guidelines

regarding the methodological structure of human science research that served to guide the present work. His six research activities which comprise the methodological structure are as follows:

1. Select a phenomenon which interests us.
2. Investigate the experience as we live it.
3. Reflect on the initial themes characterizing the phenomenon.
4. Describe the phenomenon through writing and rewriting.
5. Maintain a strong and oriented pedagogical relation to the phenomenon.
6. Balance the research context by considering parts and whole.

More specifically, we can refer to the four processes and 11 steps of van Manen's (1990) method of phenomenology that was utilized in the present study.

The first process of turning to the nature of the lived experience involved orienting to the phenomenon in question, in this case the experience of prostitution, formulating the research question, which asks what the lived experience of prostitution is, and explicates assumptions and preunderstandings that were addressed in the section on the researcher's role and bracketing. The second process, the existential investigation, involved exploring the phenomenon and generating data. For van Manen (1990) this includes using personal experience, tracing etymological sources, searching idiomatic phrases, obtaining experiential descriptions from subjects, locating experiential descriptions from other sources, and consulting phenomenological literature. The personal experience here involves my work with women who have been involved in prostitution. Tracing etymological sources—that is, researching the history and meaning of the words we use to refer to the phenomenon in question—was not a part of this study although at times a discussion was provided related to some of the terms or words used in talking about prostitution.

However, the other components were addressed in the research. Women involved in prostitution were asked to provide descriptions of their experiences, and prostitution and phenomenological literature were reviewed at length. In addition, experiential descriptions from sources other than the women involved in the study, such as from popular accounts of being in the life written by others, various websites related to prostitution and sex work, prostitution conferences I attended and colleagues who also work with women in the life, were sought out and reflected upon. The women's narratives were also examined for both content and idiomatic phrases or expressions common to prostitution and being in the life. Regarding the latter, women were asked to elaborate on what a number of terms and expressions they used in their stories meant to them. The search and analysis went beyond examining the terms of the trade, idiomatic phrases and expressions the women used, and included looking at grammatical, linguistic, and discursive elements and constructions throughout the narratives as well.

The third process, that of phenomenological reflection, directly relates to conducting the thematic analysis. For van Manen (1990) this involves uncovering thematic aspects, isolating thematic statements, composing linguistic transformations, gleaning thematic descriptions from artistic sources, and determining essential themes. In this study there was no use of artwork or art sources to uncover essential themes. Likewise, composing linguistic transformations, or writing notes and paragraphs based on my reading and other research activities, was not done either. However, the analysis involved the other components. Each audiotaped interview was listened to at least three times and the transcripts were read repeatedly and throughout the entire analysis, each time examining the overall content as well as language, making note, as indicated above, of how the women used phrases, what they said as well as how they said it, and what grammatical, linguistic, and discursive elements and constructions were evident in the narratives. According to van Manen (1990), isolating thematic statements can be done in three ways: by looking at the text as a whole, looking at phrases that stand out, or looking at every single sentence. The present study looked more at the text as a whole as well as phrases that stood out and did not use a sentence-by-sentence analysis.

After several readings a coding frame was constructed which consisted of the identified major or essential themes that appeared across the data set of all 15 narratives. From there, the major themes were examined to determine the extent to which each could contain a subset of related themes. The subset data or themes were then coded and located in the appropriate major or essential theme category. So, for example, loss was recognized as a major theme across all the women's narratives. The data was then reviewed to examine what, if any, specific examples of loss the women had experienced. The resulting subset, which could be unique to each woman and which did not have to appear across all narratives, included, for example, loss of health for some but not all women, loss of family for some but not all (in some cases loss of children, although other women retained custody of their children who stayed with family), loss of money and property for some and not all, loss of self and so on. And again, while all women spoke of "the good" of prostitution, which then became a major theme, each woman's account of what was good for her could be an individual example or subset of the major theme.

In addition to using van Manen's (1990) method of phenomenology, the data was also analyzed using what van Manen (1990) refers to as lifeworld existentials. According to van Manen (1990, p. 102) the four fundamental existentials, which consist of lived space (spatiality), lived body (corporeality), lived time (temporality) and lived other (relationality or communality), "may be seen to belong to the existential ground by way of which all human beings experience the world." Furthermore he believes that all four are helpful guides for phenomenological reflection in the research process. Spatiality is related to one's felt space, lived space, location or environment. Corporeality refers to our sense of our physical self, our actual body and our bodily presence. Temporality refers to our sense of or subjective time and lived other or relationality refers to our relationships and the lived relation we maintain with others, and how we connect to ourselves and others in the world. While the four existentials can be differentiated, they all overlap and cannot be separated. They work together to connect the dots of our life experiences, forming an intricate unity which is our lifeworld. Generally, van Manen (1990) advocates an inductive approach of being open to the thematic possibilities that can emerge from any given set of data, that is, heading into the data without having a predetermined set of categories one is looking for. However, as a means of helping the researcher reflect during phenomenological analysis, van Manen (1990) recommends consideration of the existing, or a priori categories of lifeworld existentials. While the data was analyzed in all four areas, the major themes which arose and which will be presented here are those related to the lifeworld existential of lived relation which illuminates how the women made sense of their relationships with others.

And finally, the fourth process, phenomenological writing includes attending to the speaking of the language, varying the examples, writing and rewriting. Attending to the speaking of the language requires the researcher to capture the voice and essence of the message conveyed by those whose experiences are being looked at. In addition, as van Manen (1990, p. 122) believes that we address phenomenological themes through examples, in the writing one needs to provide numerous examples so that the "invariant aspect(s) of the phenomenon itself comes into view." Once the data are analyzed, the goal is to create phenomenological descriptions that provide readers with a full and rich meaning of the lived experience in question. While not part of the analysis, the written report serves to convey the findings of the analysis. (pp. 155–161)

Research Sample and Data Sources

Unlike quantitative research, which can require large numbers of subjects, qualitative research finds smaller numbers of participants acceptable. Researchers tended to agree that as few as 10 subjects would be fine, and my committee was fine with that number. However, I wanted to interview more than that to ensure that I would have enough narratives in case some of my interviews were not usable. And indeed I did have to exclude one narrative, as it did not offer enough content to be included. Because prostitution is so stigmatized, traumatic in many cases, and illegal in all but several counties in Nevada, there was a realistic concern about finding enough participants willing to share their stories and to do so in a detailed and deep manner. As a vulnerable and somewhat underground population, this is a group of subjects who would be inaccessible to many researchers. Fortunately, because of my work with women and my connections to a number of agencies and organizations that work with this population, I did not have difficulty finding women who would speak with me. It helped that I already knew some of the women who agreed to participate and who then talked to their friends about me and encouraged them to speak to me as well. Below is the research sample and data sources excerpt from my dissertation (Sabella Monheit, 2010):

As the goal was to understand the lived experience of being involved in prostitution, the research sample consisted of women who had been directly involved in any form of prostitution. As discussed previously, there is a distinction made by some, including the women themselves, between being a sex worker or a prostituted woman. It was hoped that the study would be able to gather data from women representing both perspectives regarding prostitution and therefore attempts had been made to recruit women professing a sex work perspective as well, but none of those whom I contacted returned my calls or emails. The sample, therefore, consists exclusively of women who, while not necessarily viewing themselves as prostituted women per se, did not view themselves as sex workers.

Participant selection involved recruiting women through snowball sampling from two large American cities: one in the northeast, the other in the southwest. The first two women recruited, one from the northeast and the other from the southwest, were then asked to refer other women from their respective cities who met the study eligibility criteria. Owing to the sensitive nature of the topic, the need for confidentiality and the potential vulnerabilities and stigmatization of the women involved, there were no handouts, advertisements, brochures, public announcements, flyers or anything used which placed the recruiting of subjects in the public eye. Some of the women were enrolled in a recovery program at the time of the interviews, others had gone through one in the past, and several of the women had never sought any form of treatment at all. However, at the time of the interviews all of the women had exited prostitution and were no longer actively involved in it.

To be eligible to take part in the study each participant had to be female, had to have a current or past history of involvement in prostitution of at least a year, be over 18 years of age, and be able to give informed consent. In addition, she needed to be able to speak English well enough to describe her experiences and answer interview questions. So as not to compromise the credibility of the results, at the time of the interview a woman could not be under the influence of intoxicants or mind-altering substances or in any acute emotional distress. To determine eligibility, each participant was screened to make sure she met the participation requirements. It was recognized that there was a risk of psychological distress in asking the women to talk about their experiences as prostitution frequently involves being a victim of violence. However, efforts to minimize that in the subjects consisted of screening the women and making good faith attempts to judge that they were emotionally stable. Other attempts to minimize distress during the interviews consisted of not pushing the subjects to go beyond their comfort level, letting them know they need not talk about that which made them uncomfortable, and allowing them to stop the interview or withdraw from participation at any time. And post interview, the women not in treatment and/or in need of resources were given information to take with them if they wished about various mental health services available to them. They were also provided with my phone numbers and email addresses.

In addition, confidentiality is also of great concern as prostitution is a stigmatizing as well as illegal activity—and for many of the women, while their friends and customers know what they do, their families, especially their parents and siblings, do not. Every attempt was made to protect the participants' identities including not using their real names or identifiers in any of the study documents or data, keeping documents and tapes in a locked filing cabinet that only I had access to, keeping the list of the subjects' names cross-referenced with their pseudonyms locked in a safe that only I had access to, making sure that the tapes sent for transcription be free of any identifying information and requesting that the audiotapes be destroyed by the transcription agency once they had been transcribed. In addition, subjects were not required to sign the consent form, and were permitted to give verbal agreement to participate. Once a woman agreed to participate, either I or both of us selected a "name" to give her other than her real one. In all records, each woman is referred to only by her chosen pseudonym, including written documents and on the audio tape. For each woman, again under her pseudonym, I collected some basic information such as her age (but not date of birth), race, city of residence, marital status, number of children and level of education. In addition, the names of anyone the women referred to, including friends, relatives, bosses and the like, as well as names of cities, places or residence or other identifying information have all been changed to protect and ensure anonymity.

This study was approved by the University of Pennsylvania IRB and all guidelines and recommendations related to this work were followed to ensure the ethical treatment of the study participants and that their rights were protected. Among other things, the women were informed that they had the right to refuse to participate, the right to stop the interview at any time, the right to withdraw from the study at any time, and the right to contact me at any point with any questions or concerns they might have about the study. (pp. 129–132)

Participants

My dissertation is really the narratives of the participants. This work is truly about them, and in my Chapter Three on methodology and research design, I devoted some 10 pages to providing information and a brief biography of each participant so that the reader could come to know something about each of the women telling her story. I felt it very important to make this "introduction" in the hope of moving the reader beyond thinking of the participants as nameless and faceless participants in a study. I felt the findings would be more meaningful to readers if I could help them to understand something about who each woman was and where she was coming from. In short, what I was after was to make it clear, to the extent possible in a dissertation concerned with confidentiality, that this was a human being that I was writing about who had wants, hopes, dreams, and aspirations. I was adamant about using those pages to provide background. What follows is part of my section on participants, to give you a general idea of what I did (Sabella Monheit, 2010):

> In all, there were a total of 15 women who participated. Thirteen of those women had been involved in street-level prostitution, one had worked as a stripper, and another classified herself as an "escort of opportunity." Fourteen were American citizens and one was a citizen of an island nation, hoping to become a naturalized citizen of the United States. Twelve were of Caucasian/European background, one was Hispanic, one was of Native American background and one was of African/French descent. At the time of the interviews, the women's ages ranged from 23 to 58 years of age. The time involved in prostitution ranged from 1 to 25 years, with the age of entry from 12 to 35 years. All but two of the women also had a history of drug abuse during their time in prostitution. As it will be helpful to know something about the women who took part in the study, the following provides a bit of background information on each woman, identified by her pseudonym to protect her identity. Others as well are referred to using pseudonyms.
>
> *Marie is a 56-year-old Caucasian woman, high school graduate and former "serious" heroin addict who was involved in street-level prostitution for 10 years, beginning at the age of 35. Her entry into prostitution was directly related to her addiction and need to maintain her drug habit. Prior to her addiction and entry, she had been a married suburban housewife with children and a husband living in the northeast US with no history of drug addiction or any problems of any kind. As she stated, she was the poster woman for domestic life with a husband, three children and a white picket fence. She is now drug free and it has been 11 years since she left the life. While on the streets, her husband divorced her and she lost custody of her children, who remained with their father. She recounted that she got involved in prostitution because she saw other women doing it, thought it looked easy and she needed to make some easy money with which to buy drugs. Another woman warned her not to get involved, but she needed the money and did not listen. At first, she stated that prostitution was not all that bad, but over time, she ended up living on the streets, under bridges, and anywhere

she could lay her head down. She was at the mercy of whatever came her way. Then the arrests started as well and her life quickly spiraled out of control. Eventually for Marie being arrested was almost a welcome event as it gave her time to get cleaned up, fed, and back on her feet before she would have to hit the streets again. Eventually getting arrested and seeing information about a program for women in prostitution was the beginning of the way out and she entered treatment. While she never remarried, she has been involved in a monogamous relationship for the past 8 years with her boyfriend Arnie. She has a fulltime job as a service provider in the human services field and prides herself on keeping fit, staying active and enjoying the little things. She has been working on rebuilding the connection with her children. Like Rachel, Marie is quick, articulate and has much insight regarding her life experiences. She is also an excellent employee and devoted and loyal friend to several of the other women in the study.

*April is a 46-year-old Caucasian woman who entered prostitution at age 36 and remained in it for 6 years until she was 42. Prior to her entry she had never had a problem and was living what she considered a pretty normal life, even giving birth to a son whom she adored. However, she became addicted to drugs which drove her to commit a number of crimes. Prior to the prostitution, she had been involved in and arrested for a number of other crimes such as shop lifting and writing fraudulent checks to get money for drugs. She switched from those crimes to prostitution when she realized that the penalties for prostitution were less severe than those of her other crimes. Her life became lived out on the streets and she moved from one cheap hotel room to another, at times even sleeping in people's yards as she was frequently homeless. At one point no one would rent her a room as they found her troublesome and not worth the risk she posed of not paying for the room. She was also afraid of getting hurt because toward the end she started robbing her customers. She could not stand the sex anymore and playing the game, yet she was in desperate need of drugs, so she would take the men's money and then run off. She too was in and out of prison numerous times and it was in prison where she was given information about various treatment programs. Eventually she entered one which she completed 2 years ago. Never married, she has a son who is being raised by her mother and from whom she is estranged. In addition, the relationship with the rest of her family, including her parents, is strained. She is working on repairing that relationship with her son, of whom she lost custody once she started using drugs, and hopes that some day he will be fully back in her life. She has some college and is employed full time working with women who have experienced domestic violence as an outreach worker. She is still working on her recovery and struggles at times in her recovery, taking more steps back some days than forward. April is a beautiful, sweet and soft-spoken woman with an almost childlike gentility about her, making it hard to imagine that she was once out on the street robbing and lying to people.

*Christina, a 23 year old woman of mixed African and French descent, is the sole non-American of the group. A citizen of the island nation Martinique, she arrived in the United States to a large east coast city at the age of 14 with her father, uncle, grandfather and two brothers after her parents had separated. She started attending school in that city but dropped out of the 8th grade when her father started molesting her. As a runaway she was prey to a man who picked her up in the city and offered to help her out by taking her across the United States to the west coast, where once there, she was raped and forced into prostitution at age 17 to help pay their bills. The rape occurred because Christina was a virgin and this was the pimp's way of breaking her in for the job that awaited her. At that point her life became a living hell. She had no documents, could not speak the language well, had no education or training, had no money or family to help her and was at the mercy of men she met along the way, each one of which forced her to sell herself to make money to support him and her. She subsequently ended up in the southwest by running away from her pimp and became involved with other men, getting pregnant twice by two different men, neither one of whom wanted the baby or had plans to help support the baby. Both her children were taken from her and placed in child protection services. Each time she would call her father asking for him to send her documents so she could get legal work, he refused and said she would have to come back home if she wanted her documents. However, she had no money to do so. Her time in prostitution was a series of moving from one bad situation into another with no end in sight. Some nights Christina would pray that she would die to be released from the hell that had become her life. She was eventually arrested and spent time in prison where she was able to make arrangements to get some help. At the time of the interview, she had been out of prostitution for about 2 years, had just started in a recovery program and was working on getting her children back, getting her GED, getting therapy for the prostitution and working with immigration to be able to remain in the United States. She is not working as she is in treatment fulltime. (pp. 132–137)

INSTITUTIONAL REVIEW BOARD (IRB)

I found myself amused by the fact that the Internal Revenue Service (IRS) and institutional review board (IRB) differ by only one letter. While we can choose our chair and our committee, forget about having any control in this area. I had a few moments of panic when dealing with the IRB at my institution. For them, the business of review and dealing with all that this entails is business as usual, but for novice researchers and green doctoral students, that is not the case. They had issues about my interviewing the women and wanted me to apply for a higher level of approval as this was a population who "might be engaged" in criminal activity. Luckily I prevailed, as to do what they wanted me to do would have delayed my getting started on interviews by possibly months, plus it was not necessary. You will definitely need to be prepared for the IRB to make recommendations and requests regarding a number of things from minor to major. Most of their feedback to me focused on sentence wording, which was easy to address as they provided the exact wording they wanted me to use, so all I had to do was change my wording to theirs. The majority of their suggestions were reasonable, but I took exception to one in particular. They gave me trouble over using the term "in the life," saying that it could refer to a number of things. I was asked to remove it, but I did not. I found that request ridiculous, as that is the term that is frequently used and widely known when speaking about prostitution. Aside from wording issues, my other complaint centers on their dropping the ball when I was kept waiting for the final approval decision. It turned out that the woman in the office who had been working with me left for vacation—without telling me and without putting an away message up on her e-mail account. My e-mails to her went unanswered, and it was only after 2 weeks of waiting on my end to hear back from her that I finally summoned up the courage—as I certainly did not want to annoy anyone in the IRB office—to e-mail someone else in the office to see what was going on. At that point I was told that the woman was on vacation, but her colleague did follow up for me. But that caused a delay of several weeks, which, although not the end of the world, came close to my having to change my travel plans to travel out of state to interview women.

As mentioned earlier, confidentiality was rightfully of the utmost importance to the women, the IRB, and me, and I actually bought a safe that only I had access to in which to store the tapes and transcriptions. I also had another smaller lock box that contained the women's real names cross referenced with their pseudonyms. Also, because all of the women had at least one street or working name while they were out there, I went as far as to not even use their working or street names in the interviews, lest they be identified through that name. The women were asked to use another street name in their accounts. A number of the women were friends with each other and knew that they were all being interviewed by me, but I made it clear to everyone that, friends or not, I would not acknowledge that fact, even though we all knew it to be the case.

Setting

I interviewed the women in a variety of settings. Some of the women with whom I spoke were in a recovery program, and I requested and was granted permission to interview them at the program's facilities in a room that was private. Of course, other women living there saw me coming in but were not given details about why I was there. It helped that the arrangements for volunteers had been made ahead of time so the women who had agreed to participate were supposedly the only ones who knew why I was there, unless of course they shared that information with others in the house, which was something that I had no control over. This involved sending the agency a letter requesting permission to speak with women in the program and a copy of the IRB approval form, which detailed what I wanted to do. They gave permission and requested that I conduct the interviews on site. This was actually helpful, as I then did not have to look for an appropriate interview setting on my own.

In addition to a "formalized" setting of a recovery program, I also interviewed some women at their homes and a few, who worked in women's support services, asked that I interview them at work, which their employers permitted. There too I was given a private space with a door that closed and where no one could overhear us or enter without our knowledge. And finally, two interviews were conducted in my rental car, as one woman took her lunch hour while at work to meet with me and another had children at home and did not want to share her story in their presence. She had to wait until her husband got home from work in the evening so he could watch the kids while we met. At that hour, the car was the most convenient place to meet. There were no problems in any of the settings, as fortunately they all afforded comfort and privacy, although the car interviews started to get a bit uncomfortable physically after an hour. It was important that the women felt comfortable during the interview, so a setting that fostered this feeling for them, protected their privacy and confidentiality, and had limited distractions was essential. Likewise, having a space and setting that provided us with as much time for the interview as needed was also crucial, especially because I did not establish a set start and stop time across the board and hoped that each woman would have and take whatever time she needed to share her story.

Data Collection Procedures and Ethical Considerations

This was one of the best parts of the process. After months of planning, getting approval from various gatekeepers, meeting with my chair, lining up participants, making travel arrangements, and making sure that I had plenty of batteries for the tape recorders, it was now "go time." I was actually going to sit down with the women and begin collecting their narratives. I was thrilled, as it meant that I was finally at the threshold and poised to get to the heart of the matter. The following excerpt is from Chapter 3: Methodology and Research Design, and it addresses data collection and procedure (Sabella Monheit, 2010).

According to Boyd (2001) and Creswell (1998) two to ten subjects is a large enough number to reach saturation when doing phenomenological research. I had originally decided on interviewing 10 participants, but 15 volunteered. Upon meeting the women and determining that all 15 met the criteria, I then interviewed everyone who wanted to participate. As mentioned above, the women were recruited from two major American cities through snowballing. Maxwell (2005) details four points to consider related to method in doing qualitative research. The two relevant here speak of how, among other things, participants are selected and the relationships that the researcher then establishes with participants in the study. As mentioned previously, women who met the established criteria related to the study were invited to participate. Most important, as the research question revolved around the lived experience of prostitution, all participants had to have been involved in some form of prostitution at some point in their life for at least a year. Initially I did not rule out women who were still involved in prostitution and would have accepted someone still in the life as a study participant. However, in the end all of the women recruited had exited prostitution. A woman also had to be of age, be willing to share her experiences with me and not be under the influence. To maintain some level of objectivity I chose not to recruit women with whom I had either a professional or closely personal relationship, which eliminated all the women I had worked with in the groups I conduct in Philadelphia. Participants were recruited through snowballing wherein I contacted a woman in each of the two cities where the interviews were conducted and they in turn connected me with women they knew via word of mouth. An equally important factor as per Maxwell (2005) focuses on the relationships established with the participants in the study. As will be discussed in more detail in Chapter 7, I was acquainted with seven of the study participants through previous contact I had with them several years prior to conducting this research when I was working on another project. However, I knew the women as acquaintances in passing and was on friendly terms with them. The women, I believe, thought well of me and when they were told that I wanted to interview women involved in prostitution for my dissertation, they agreed to do so because of our favorable prior contacts. I believe the women felt comfortable in speaking with me and they all knew of my background as a nurse and someone working in the field. However, there were eight women I had never met whom I interviewed, but who had heard about me from those who did. Undoubtedly the relationship, whether prior or new, had the potential to impact upon how the women related their experiences to me, how they viewed me, and how they positioned themselves in our interaction. How the women viewed me and wanted me to view them and how they positioned themselves in our interaction is relevant regarding the findings and the implications of those findings.

If a woman expressed interest in participating, I spoke to her either in person or over the phone to give her some general background information about the research and answer any questions she had at the time. My contact information was provided to her so she could contact me at any time and an appointment was made to then meet in person. At that time I also shared with the women my being a doctoral candidate/researcher in addition to being a mental health nurse involved in working with women involved in prostitution in Philadelphia, and that the information gathered would be used in both my dissertation as well as in helping to inform treatment of other women in and/or leaving prostitution.

Once I was face to face with a woman, I requested permission to speak to her about the study, determined her eligibility to take part in the study, and provided her a copy of the informed consent to read over and keep, stressing to her that she had the right to not participate if she so chose after reading through the consent form. I explained in more detail what the study was about, its purpose, procedure, potential risks and benefits, her right to withdraw at any time, and conditions of confidentiality, and I answered all her questions. At that point, I gave her the option of thinking it over and scheduling the interview for a later date. All of the women declined this option and wanted to begin the interview at our initial meeting. As I either personally knew the women or they had been contacted by someone they knew who knew me as well and who vouched for my integrity, I believe that there was a certain element of trust going into this that was beneficial to the process. I informed each woman that she did not need to sign the consent form and that by agreeing to be taped she was giving her consent to participate.

The interviews were all conducted in locations and settings of the women's choice, based on where they felt most comfortable, including their homes, private offices I had access to, and in two cases, in my car. The interviews, which were audiotaped, consisted of two parts. In the first half of the interview each woman was asked to share with me what her experience in prostitution was like for her. In addition to that interview question, in the second half of the interview each woman was asked to elaborate on a number of other things based on what she had or had not shared in telling her story during the first part of the interview. A pilot study had been conducted in the spring of 2009 with two women who were interviewed and asked to share their narratives with me about what their experiences in prostitution had been like for them. While the women did indeed talk about their experiences in prostitution, they focused more on what they did than on the nature of the lived experience and what the experience meant and how it felt to them. Based on the outcomes and findings of that pilot study, this time around it was stressed to the participants that they were being asked to talk about what the experience was like for them and not necessarily what they did while involved in prostitution. In addition, as a result of the pilot study, a number of possible follow-up prompts or questions based on findings which emerged from those interviews were developed. Those prompts, related to the existing research question regarding the lived experience, were viewed as potentially helpful in excavating and uncovering deeper meaning related to the present research question and getting the most out of the interviews. They were brought into each interview and asked on an as-needed basis depending on what the woman had shared during the first half of her interview.

During the first part of the interviews each woman was asked to describe and share with me her lived experience of what it was like for her to be involved in prostitution. She was asked the following question: Could you please share with me and talk to me about what it was like for you to be involved in prostitution? Each woman was told she could speak for as little or long as she wished and that she did not have to detail anything that would cause her discomfort. Questions during the first part of the interview were asked sparingly by me and only for clarification or elaboration purposes. During this part of the interview I also jotted down some notes highlighting areas I wanted to address in more detail with the woman after she had completed telling her story based on what she had shared with me in the first half of the interview. Often these notes were related to the possible prompts mentioned above and listed below. After having shared her experiences and telling her story about what the experience had been like for her, each woman was offered the chance to take a break. The interview then continued to the second part, in which questions were asked of the women related to areas they had addressed or touched upon during the first part which I wanted to explore further with them. The questions asked of the women in the second part of the interview depended on what they had or had not addressed in the first part and therefore not all of the questions were asked. The list served only as a possible guideline. The list of possible scripted questions taken into the interviews is provided below:

- Tell me how you became involved in prostitution.
- What kept you involved in prostitution?
- How would you complete this sentence: I am ….
- How would you complete this sentence: Prostitutes are/Prostitution is ….
- Could you share with me who you are/how you identify yourself now, before and after your experience in prostitution?
- Tell me how you came to leave prostitution (if the woman is no longer involved in prostitution).
- Would you like to leave prostitution (if she is still involved)?
- What keeps you/kept you in the life?
- What is something you'd like everyone to know about you?
- What is something you'd like everyone to know about prostitutes/prostitution/being in the life?
- Who were you growing up, while in prostitution, and who you are now?
- What do you think of other women in the life?
- What do you think of women who aren't in the life?
- What is your street/working name?
- Who are/were you when you're using a street or working name (which will not be mentioned)?
- How do you feel about what you do/did?
- How do you react when people talk about prostitutes?

- What do you think about what people say about prostitutes/ prostitution?
- What do you think would be helpful for people who work with women involved in prostitution to know about the women and how to help them?
- What, if any, were the positive, negative and neutral aspects of being in prostitution for you?

While Seidman (1998) argues for conducting a series of three interviews which focus on the respondent's life history in the first interview, the respondent's current experience in the second, and the subject's understanding of those experiences in the final interview, owing to the lifestyle and availability of women involved in prostitution, requesting to meet three times was believed to put an undue burden on the women, and even asking to meet twice was not possible for most of the women. In addition, conducting multiple interviews would have required extensive and repeated travel to the sites for the researcher. Therefore, all data was collected at the first and only interview, which was audiotaped, and women were given the option of contacting me via phone or email should they wish to add anything else or make changes.

As Elliott (2005) states, many suggest that 90 minutes is the optimum amount of time for a qualitative research interview. While not adhering to a specific timetable, the interview length was left up to each woman depending on how long she wished to speak for and how much she wished to share. Interview times ranged from approximately 60 minutes to a little more than 90 minutes. The tapes were then sent out for transcription and the transcripts were subsequently analyzed as discussed below. At the end of the interview, each woman not in treatment or wishing the information was given information regarding treatment resources in her area should she decide to seek any form of support and/or help. All women also received a $30 gift card to a local department store to thank her for her time. Receiving financial rewards for being in such studies is common practice and would help to make up for money lost for not working while being interviewed. In her work with prostitutes, Boynton (2002) recommends that whenever possible, participants should receive payment. The women were also given my card with a contact email and phone number in case they wished to add anything later or change their mind about being involved in the research and having their narrative included in the data. (pp. 143–149)

I was also highly cognizant of what I was asking the women to do and wanted to make sure I included a statement on ethical considerations. Here is that excerpt (Sabella Monheit, 2010):

Violence is often a part of prostitution and for that reason it was not unexpected that talking about her experiences in the life would cause the woman to discuss some unpleasant and hurtful aspects of those experiences. Should any woman have evidenced signs of trauma during or after the interview, the interview would have been halted and the woman provided with appropriate mental health intervention. At no time during any of the interviews under any circumstances was a woman forced or encouraged to speak about something she did not want to. In 2005, I began interviewing women about their involvement in prostitution and have done so since then both professionally to counsel as well as to collect data used in designing the mental health treatment program for Dawn's Place. As a mental health professional, I have experience and knowledge in working with prostituted women and hearing their stories in a professional, ethical, and responsible manner.

As the focus of this research relies on input from vulnerable populations, it is paramount that a number of factors be considered throughout to protect the women's well-being in addition to the above. In her work on working with vulnerable populations, among which she includes prostitutes, Liamputtong (2007) addresses a number of important issues for what she calls the sensitive researcher to keep in mind. Among them are the morality of the research, ethical issues such as informed consent, confidentiality, and participant safety, and ways to build trust and establish rapport with one's participants. Likewise, a number of other researchers working specifically with prostitutes offer sound advice on some of the methodological and ethical issues and challenges facing those researching this population (Boynton, 2002; Melrose, 2002; Shaver, 2005). Among the various issues are the concern that the women are involved in a criminal activity, the risk of physical harm and violence to the pimp-controlled women, researchers needing to process some of their own upsetting experiences in hearing the women's stories, and how to successfully terminate the relationship once the research is over. Every precaution and all necessary steps were taken to protect and guard the safety, well-being, dignity, and confidentiality of those involved in this study, including that of the researcher. One of the biggest concerns relates to the woman signing her real name on the consent form. As mentioned earlier, no woman was required to do so. Her consent was verbally provided and implied as we began taping the interview. (pp. 149–150)

Timeline

"The best dissertation is a done dissertation" was my mantra, although not initially. Initially there was always one more article to read or one more chapter in a book to look over. It was as if some divine piece of wisdom would be hidden deep inside someone else's work and that I would be the poorer for not having discovered that all-important piece of knowledge and information that would be the key to my having a dissertation that was the mother of all dissertations. Either that or reading one more of anything was a diversionary tactic to avoid getting to the task at hand: the actual writing. Or perhaps it was a combination of the two. I also realized that I had to stop accepting offers to teach interesting and challenging courses in addition to my full-time job. Once I stopped the sideshow events, academic and other-wise, and avoidance tactics—which did take some time, I'll admit—I started to live the mantra and made the dissertation my focus. I set aside regular and set times every week to work on it and learned to use it to my advantage by getting out of things I neither wanted nor had to do or attend. I had my proposal hearing in December 2009, submitted to the IRB in January 2010, collected data in March and April, and defended and passed in October of 2010. It took less than a year and this on top of a new full-time faculty posi-tion on a 12-month schedule and 3 children in college. My advice: The best dissertation is a done dissertation!

Data Analysis

While data collection for me was comparable to unwrapping a present, data analysis was akin to taking the gift out of the box to see what I had been given. It was getting the answers to the questions that I wanted answers to. There I was surrounded by an unimaginable amount of information and a number of words, and it was time to sort through all of that, much like an archaeologist, to see what treasures my search might yield. This was what it was all about. While interviewing the women I had heard their words, but at this juncture, thanks to the magic of recording and transcription, I had the luxury of sitting back and savoring their stories. I could shut everything out and immerse myself in their words and worlds, past, present, and future.

I gave myself up to them as their words took me through their journey to places I could not go on my own and to a place of richer and deeper understanding. It was frustrating at times, and it did involve complete focus and attention, as well as revisiting their narratives over and over, even at times to the point of oversaturation. But when I found myself feeling too immersed and blurry-headed, I took a break and came back refreshed.

As mentioned previously, my background, aside from mental health nursing, involves training in and study of language—among other things, how we acquire or learn it, how we use it in society, how it is structured, and how we tell stories that help us make sense of our lives and experiences. My framework for the analysis is based on examining the women's narratives and in this excerpt I detail what that means, and what I did (Sabella Monheit, 2010):

> Narrative may be used in the investigation of a variety of research questions both as a means of obtaining the data and as the end or object of research in and of itself. As the present research analyzes narratives to get to the heart of the phenomenon and there is overlap between narrative and phenomenology, I believe it important to provide some background information regarding analysis. In what follows below I offer a brief and general overview regarding various perspectives on analyzing narratives before focusing on the method and framework used in this study.
>
> Narrative analysis is defined as a method of qualitative research whereby the researcher reads or listens to the subjects' stories and attempts to understand the connections between the experiences described by the individuals and their social framework. Daiute and Lightfoot (2004) conceptualize narrative analysis as a mode of inquiry based upon narrative being a root metaphor, a genre and a discourse.
>
> According to McLeod (2001), the development of a narrative approach to analyzing interview data can be largely attributed to Elliot Mishler (1986a, 1986b) and the subsequent work of his former student Catherine Riessman (1993). McLeod (2001) views narrative analysis as an approach that combines a discursive emphasis on the construction of meaning through talk and language with a humanistic image of the narrator as a self-aware agent seeking meaning, control and fulfillment in life.
>
> In health care, particularly in behavioral health, narratives are believed to assist in recovery (Charon, 2007; Davidson, 2003; Lysaker & Buck, 2006). However, in spite of the popularity of narrative within numerous fields, Elliott (2005) informs us that there is no definitive

definition of narrative analysis. Although there are numerous suggestions explaining how one can perform an analysis of literary text, she points out that there is no standard approach, no single method, nor any list of procedures that represent the narrative method of analysis, and she quotes Mishler (1995, p. 88) who states that there is a state of near anarchy in the field with regard to a narrative method of analysis, a state of affairs agreed upon by others as well (Baumgartner, 2000; McLeod, 2001).

Within the anarchy, however, there are a number of proposed frameworks for classifying methods of narrative analysis. According to Lieblich et al. (1998), narrative materials can be analyzed for, among other things, content, structure, speech style, affective characteristics, motives, attitudes, and beliefs of the narrator. McAdams (1993) argues that important concepts to identify in the analysis consist of narrative tone, imagery, and themes. Clearly there is no single set of guidelines for how to proceed and what to analyze (Riessman, 1993).

According to Baumgartner (2000), the most common types of narrative analysis are psychological, biographic and linguistic. Related most closely to the present study are the psychological methods of analysis, which focus on the meaning people create through the words they use and the stories they tell and which are less concerned with linguistic forms and structure. Biographic analysis takes into account the role of society in helping to create the individuals' narratives (Denzin, 1989). And the linguistic approach, such as that of Labov and Waletzky's (1967/1997) frequently cited structuralist technique, breaks narrative down into various linguistic structures and clauses. Mishler (1995), in his typology of narrative analysis, offers a framework for analysis based on the language functions of meaning, structure, and interactional context. Hiles (2007) argues that one cannot separate form from content. In doing narrative analysis, he maintains that one must pay attention to both the what and the how of the telling, a position that he realizes is in opposition to many of the approaches to narrative analysis. While the above approaches to analysis are presented as distinct means to an end, I believe it important to acknowledge that the psychological content of a narrative has the potential to inform the linguistic/discursive form of the narrative and likewise, the linguistic/discursive form can impact the psychological content of the narrative. Narrative exists neither in a vacuum nor completely independent of what is going on around it. The interactional context as well has a bearing upon what gets said, how it gets said, why it gets said, and even what does not get spoken of and why. The interactional context, linguistic/discursive form, and psychological content are all intertwined and overlap, and at times are not so easily teased apart in analysis.

Aside from psychological, biographic, and linguistic approaches mentioned above there are a number of other analytic approaches. Braun and Clarke (2006) describe thematic analysis as a method of analyzing narratives. Although they state that there is no clear agreement regarding exactly what thematic analysis is, they define it as a method of identifying, analyzing, and reporting patterns or themes within the data, as was the case in the present study which looked to identify, describe and analyze themes that emerged in the women's narratives. Murray (2000) informs us that in health psychology, health and illness narratives can be analyzed at four different levels: personal, interpersonal, positional and societal. Simply stated, analysis at the personal level relates to the stories that people tell about their own health and illness and how their narratives portray their lived experience of such. Analysis at an interpersonal level views narrative as being coauthored in a dialog with others. Positional analysis takes into account the differences in social position between the narrator and listener and the societal level of analysis takes into account how narratives are representative of socially shared stories shared by certain communities or groups. Lieblich and colleagues (1998) classify types of narrative analysis depending on whether one focuses on form or content, and on the entire narrative (holistic) as opposed to a specific event (categorical) within the narrative. Their four proposed modes of analysis include holistic content, holistic form, categorical content and categorical form. As mentioned earlier, the present study takes into account the content of the woman's entire narrative, thereby using a holistic-content mode of analysis.

With regard to narrative and its analysis, Riessman (1993, 2008) theorizes the research process as consisting of five levels of representation. While not the exact approach used in the current study as the structure of the narrative was not a main focus, the steps are very similar to what was done here and what van Manen (1990) proposes, making it clear that in spite of different approaches, there is overlap among them. The first level involves the narrator at some point attending to what will be contained in the narrative, eventually telling the story. The researcher's work at level two is to facilitate the telling of the narrative during the interview. Once in receipt of the story, which has been recorded, analysis begins as the researcher transcribes the data, entering level three. The fourth level involves the researcher analyzing the transcript, making numerous decisions about how to proceed and what to include, and looking for what she needs to interpret meaning and construct a meta-story about what happened. The final level involves the reader encountering the written report. For Riessman (2008), transcribing and analyzing are closely related and not easily distinguished. Performing close and repeated listening in conjunction with methodic transcription often leads to insights which Riessman (1993) believes shape how the narrative is represented in the text. She states that she discourages students from entering into narrative research with hard and fixed ideas and research questions because analytic induction causes new questions to emerge and prior ones to change. While acknowledging the many ways to analyze the interview data, Riessman (1993, 2008) recommends beginning with analyzing the structure of the narrative before examining the meaning and asking such questions related to how the narrative is organized and why the narrator chose to develop her narrative in the way she has. She also acknowledges that thematic analysis is the most common approach in narrative analysis, which she also views as compatible to phenomenology and hermeneutics. Here again the link is made between phenomenology and narrative. (pp. 150–155)

FINDINGS

In the end, this is what it's all about: What did I learn from this research that I did not know before? What are the outcomes? What was discovered? What are the findings? Yes, we go through this process because it is a requirement, but how empty and meaningless this would be if that were all there was to it. And I suppose there are some who indeed just go through the motions to get to the desired prize. But I am sure that most of us hope to come away from an expedition of this kind with some answers and discoveries that are of value and that bring about positive effects in some areas. While involved in the process, I did experience some moments when I hoped that I would "find" something of value and not come away empty-handed, and I suppose that is not an uncommon fear among researchers, especially novices. There is no guarantee that we will always find something when we go looking for it. However, once the analysis was completed, I was rewarded with a number of rich and what I thought of as valuable findings. As mentioned earlier, my dissertation consisted of seven chapters, three of which focused on findings. Chapter 4: In the Life, shared findings related to how the women first became involved in prostitution, what their first experience was like, why they stayed, and how they exited. Chapter 5: The Good, the Bad and the Ugly, which I found especially interesting, focused on what the women viewed as the good, the bad, and the ugly aspects of prostitution. Chapter 6, Identity, Agency and Lived Relation, examined a number of issues related to self and public identity, their sense of their own agency, and a variety of relationships they had, including with men and others in their lives. There was much to be discovered. I refer you to the actual dissertation if you would like to know more, but in the following sections, I would like to share some of the content from those chapters with you (Sabella Monheit, 2010). It is in these chapters that the women's voices can be heard, and even though you have not been introduced to all of them, I believe you will see how powerful some of their comments and reflections are.

Chapter 4: In the Life

> This chapter and those that follow address a number of themes that emerged based on what the women shared about their experiences of being in the life in their narratives. In this chapter, I will address a number of important themes that emerged around why the women entered prostitution, what their first experience in it was like, why they stayed in it, and how they came to leave. In terms of themes identified as to why they entered prostitution, the majority of women understood their entrance as being connected to needing drugs and/or money, material things, and wanting to feel a sense of love and belonging. For some women, there were several reasons and even for those who had articulated a very clear reason, they were still struggling to make sense of why they had taken the path they did. With regard to the women's accounts of how their first time happened, the themes of agency and responsibility, and how the women characterized their level of participation related to their initiation into the life are addressed as well as the themes of force and grooming, and chance and accident. Likewise, in examining the women's accounts of why they remained involved in prostitution, the themes of agency and empowerment related to their sense of getting stuck are addressed as are the secondary gains or benefits they described receiving while involved in prostitution. And finally, in terms of how the women understood and narrated their exiting the life, I examine the theme of exit by arrest as well as their perceptions of how the bad began to outweigh the good, again connecting those themes to the women's sense of agency, responsibility, and power. (p. 164)

This excerpt in the chapter talks about getting involved in prostitution by chance and accident (Sabella Monheit, 2010):

Chance and Accident

For a number of women, their accounts regarding their entry into prostitution rely on the notion of things happening to them by chance or accident, with their role, at least initially, that of bystander just minding their own business out in public. In their narratives, the women described no purposeful action or human agency on their part that created the situation that invited them into prostitution. Rather, the situation seemed to have arisen naturally and out of someone else's agency and desire, but not theirs. However, once the request had been issued, the women do acknowledge their responsibility in accepting and acting upon the invitation put forth to them. In the examples that follow, the women describe how they required no time at all to consider the invitation, acting upon it immediately to provide a sexual service for money. April, battling a drug addiction at the time, had not previously considered getting involved in prostitution. Homeless and just released from jail where she had served time for retail theft, she was walking along looking for someplace to get high when she was invited to try prostitution for the first time by a man driving along who pulled up to her. She quickly realized that she had found a better way to get money than stealing and breaking and entering. Although describing her entrance as something that "kinda happened by accident" allowed her to distance herself from appearing to have actively sought out prostitution and sold herself for money, she is clear that "I did it" and acknowledges embracing wholeheartedly the prospect of being involved in prostitution:

> When I first did it, it kinda happened by accident. Um, I was walking down the street. This guy pulled up beside me and he asked if I was working. And I remember saying to him, like, no, I don't have a job, you know. I didn't understand. And he saw that I didn't get it. And he just said, "Do you want a ride?" My feet are—you know—I mean if I can get to where I was going faster to get this drug in me faster and not feel this pain. Well, during the ride he ended up offering me a whole bunch of money for something pretty simple. And I did it. He gave me all the money he promised me plus some more, got me something to eat and dropped me off right at the drug house. And I thought "Wow! This is my new crime." (pp. 177–178)

Chapter Five: The Good, The Bad, and The Ugly

This chapter I found very interesting and it challenged the all-good or all-bad discourse often recited in relation to prostitution. The following is an introduction to the chapter with some excerpts from various sections within Chapter Five (Sabella Monheit, 2010):

> As has been mentioned previously, while the public holds and entertains various perspectives regarding numerous aspects of prostitution, almost everyone, regardless of their position on the subject, agrees that there are indeed negative aspects to being involved in prostitution. For example, whether it is legal or not, or whether one views prostitution as morally right or wrong, or as the right or not of every woman to decide what to do with her body, few would deny that there is an element of violence that confronts all "working women" and few would deny the stigma that surrounds selling sex. That there are bad and ugly elements to contend with comes as no surprise, and indeed, much of what the women in this study had to say about and make sense of their being involved in prostitution details some of the specifics of what was bad and ugly about it for them. But aside from the negative, the women also spoke of some of the good and what they got out of their experience in prostitution both at the time they were involved in it as well as when they walked away. In all cases, the women were not originally asked to talk about the good, bad, and ugly of their life in the life. The original question posed to them asked them to describe and characterize their involvement in prostitution and to talk about what the experience was like for them. However, in the second part of the interview, follow-up questions regarding what they had said about the good, bad, and ugly were asked when necessary to further excavate and mine what they had said earlier. An analysis of the women's narratives made it clear that there were three major categories to be examined: the good, the bad, and the ugly. In addition, a number of themes emerged that could be placed into each category. As phenomenology seeks to understand the meaning, description, and characterizations that those living a certain experience assign to that experience, the present study examines how the women in this study did so. In essence, in their narratives the women characterized their lived prostitution experience as a mix of things that ranged from being positive and/or beneficial at one end of the continuum to being

traumatic and horrific at the other end, as well as a number of other things in between. In short, for many of the women their experiences in prostitution contained elements of both paradox and contradiction, for to borrow a line from Dickens, it was a mix of both the best of times and the worst of times.

This chapter presents what the women had to say about and how they made sense of what they perceived to be the positive and negative aspects of their time and experiences in prostitution and how they were able to integrate and incorporate, what appears to be, at times, the paradoxical and contradictory nature of prostitution. What they found to be good is presented first followed by the categories of the bad and ugly aspects of their involvement in prostitution. Because not much has been written about or shared in the literature that addresses what women perceive to be beneficial or positive about their experience in prostitution, the women's statements about that aspect of their experience in prostitution are shared in greater detail here in order to provide the reader with a deeper understanding of the women's perspectives and sense making. It is important to note that while the good, the bad, and the ugly are presented as separate categories of the women's experiences, while they are relative, different, and distinct, they do work together to form the whole of the lived experience. It should also be noted that what each woman viewed as good, bad, or ugly was subject to change, depending on her situation and vantage point at the time, something which a number of women pointed out in their interviews. (pp. 197–198)

Below we see what three women said that was related to their perception of the "good" they experienced while in the life (Sabella Monheit, 2010):

If a woman experienced one good thing about prostitution, it usually followed that she experienced a number of other good things as well. No woman in this study acknowledged one and only one positive aspect or benefit of being involved in prostitution and throughout their narratives the women spoke of a number of benefits and things they enjoyed during the course of their involvement. April explained that it wasn't so bad "out there" or she would not have stayed out there for as long as she did. Her comments reveal that there were a number of things she found attractive at the time regarding her involvement in prostitution, including being wanted, getting attention and money, being able to escape from herself, feeling powerful and in control, the excitement of the unknown, and the adrenaline rush of living life on the edge. However, the "good" had a relatively short shelf life and, as was the case with the other women, over time the good started to expire and turn bad. While in the life, she was well aware that eventually there would be more bad than good. And from where she is today, April looked back and realized that while some of these things are good, like having money, feeling wanted, and having power, she can find other ways to achieve them than through prostitution. Below she shares what some of positive aspects of prostitution were for her (p. 202):

> I felt powerful. I felt wanted. I felt like I was getting attention. This [prostitution] worked better for me [compared to her other crimes] because, it was, it was kinda like being an actress for a little amount of time. And I wanted to—I didn't want to be myself anyway, you know. So it was nice for me to play somebody else. There, the money was good. The amount of time you had to spend with one person for the amount of money you made was incredible, you know. You could have somebody in and out of your room in 10 minutes very happy and have a pocketful of money. I mean *it was—that—that* was a very powerful feeling. There was just an adrenaline rush and a feeling of a feel-good from setting up the transaction to getting the money. Kinda like a sale, like a car salesman selling a car or something like that. You don't have to wait for a paycheck. Sometimes it was exciting because you never know what's going to happen next. You know, it's that element of surprise, you know. That excitement and adrenaline rush feeling that you get from just being totally vulnerable and just being, or thinking you're in control. I mean, it's just so crazy. (p. 203)

Diana also shared a number of things she enjoyed related to her involvement in prostitution, including getting money, feeling wanted and loved, getting attention, being in control, and experiencing the thrill of doing something illegal without getting caught:

> I served a lot of time on the street. It was about money. It was about making money, it was about being wanted by others, it was about having the attention. It was, um, it was a high being

out there. It was excitement. Doing certain acts in the car and not being caught. Just being, kind of having this sneaky motivation and, um, getting away with it. Um, making the money. It's a high just as it is using drugs or drinking alcohol. It's a thrill. I enjoyed being around people. I enjoyed, um, having some of those guys take me out and spend money on me. I enjoyed getting my way. I mean I've had men take me on, uh, clothing, and take me out and just buy me clothing, shopping sprees. I've had a gentleman buy me a car. I've, you know, just been able to get what I wanted, um, out of using them. And I think that you know, that was exciting. That was the good. And, um, I've even, even felt loved by, um, some of the men. It seemed like, you know, I was loved. I may have been full of bologna, but, um, it sure felt like it at the time. (p. 203)

In Angelica's account detailing her view of the positive of her experience in prostitution, she hits upon a number of themes common across the other women's narratives including the thrill of the hunt, making big money, staying high, being in control, experiencing fun and excitement, and having good sex. At least initially for Angelica, there was a honeymoon period where the good outweighed the bad and where she was not even ready to consider the possibility of the problems that might be awaiting her down the road:

Getting ready to go out and score that big money, and then being able to—you know, and that's what was fun and exciting about it, you know. Getting that big-dollar trick and doing all those things, and being able to stay high. And it just, for me, that fun and excitement was enough to keep my mind occupied. And then I discovered it was about the control because I felt that I was in such control over the situation and what happened. There was too much excitement and feel-good. Not for a minute did I consider that there would be any kind of danger. I didn't think about any of that because that feel-good, that power, that control, that money, all that stuff that it gave me far outweighed any of the negative consequences in my mind at that time. Um, and yeah, I met some people that I really liked, even some tricks that were, you know, really okay people too, you know—and yeah, sometimes the sex was really good, especially when you're on drugs. You know what I mean? (pp. 203–204)

But there was also bad. Below Marie describes how her life spiraled out
of control while she was on the streets:

> Prostitution becomes a really lonely, ugly experience. I think it's
> gradual. I think it was gradual. I think that, um, uh, you see people
> around you die. Um, you see people that were one way and then
> like all of a sudden they're like different people. And you see your-
> self in others. You see the decline. You do things like out of sheer
> desperation that are like really humiliating. I mean they really are.
> You laugh about it with your friends, but the reality is that it's
> pathetic. The last years on the street were really ugly. I stopped
> lying to myself. I just was like a dead person—the walking dead,
> like a zombie, you know? You go out and you do what you gotta
> do. If you get to that place where you really believe there's no
> purpose in your life, it makes it a real easy decision [to commit sui-
> cide]. And that's a really hard place and I wouldn't wish that place
> on my worst enemy. I lived like that for years, you know? I mean
> seven years is a long time to live in that place. (p. 227)

Violence was a common theme related to the "bad." Below Diana and
then Nicole share their experiences:

> The things that turned it [prostitution] into a nightmare is not
> everybody, uh, that picked you up was nice. Not everybody that
> picked you up, um, respected you. I've been raped. I've been
> robbed. I've been held at gunpoint. I've been almost strangled to
> death. Um, uh, I, I, I've been through some, um, really horrific,
> uh, times. Um, I've fell asleep in cars and been handcuffed and
> taken places. Um, it's, um, it's not really—it's not really what it's
> cracked up to be. I know the one time when I was almost stran-
> gled to death. I had no idea that this man was capable of putting
> something around my neck, and, um, was willing to strangle me.
> And I had no vibes. I, I didn't know. And, uh, I know that my
> head went numb and all I could think was, "God, please let me
> say something." And I, I was 6 months pregnant at the time, and
> I said, "Please, I'm pregnant," and he let go of whatever he had
> around my neck, and said, "Oh, god, why didn't you tell me?"
> And he reached over, he opened the door and just told me to get
> out. And I'll never forget that, you know. It was like he could've
> just finished me, but instead he didn't. (p. 249)

I could be beat up, tore up. I remember one time my ribs were kicked and I couldn't even hardly walk down the street. But I couldn't [think about having gotten beaten] because it was too painful, you know, or they took the money back, or you know. And then I would be going, "Ah, shoot. What am I gonna do now?" And so the only solution I have is—because I really gotta get high. I gotta numb this pain physically, mentally, emotionally, spiritually. I can remember just walking up and down the street, up and down the street. I can remember just never ending. I would walk for hours and hours and hours. Uh, I wouldn't, until I could turn a date I wouldn't eat. Um, maybe I'd smoke a couple cigarettes. I obviously didn't have any drugs because I'm out there because I need more money. Um, just the pain, the hurt, the tired. (p. 250)

Chapter 6: Identity, Agency, and Lived Relation

The following text is the introduction to Chapter 6 followed by various excerpts related to identity and relations (Sabella Monheit, 2010):

Chapter 6 addresses the themes that emerged in the women's narratives related to the constructs of identity and agency as well as van Manen's (1990) lifeworld existential of lived relation. I begin with a brief introduction providing information and background about the many ways of defining and approaching the study of identity. I then present findings related to identity and stigma, how the women self-identified, the connection between identity and morality, how others identified the women, and how they described their prostitution identity. In addition, I provide findings regarding what the women had to say related to their deciding to use street names or not and of their having a lost or abandoned identity, resulting in their not having a sense of who they are. The subsequent section offers background information related to the construct of personal agency and examines how the women made sense of their level of agency and who they felt really had control and provided for them in the life. Finally, I present findings related to van Manen's (1990) lifeworld existential of lived relation, which the women addressed in their narratives, and the important role that relationships played in their lives. (p. 257)

Identity and how the women felt the public viewed them was something a number of women addressed in their narratives. Below Marie challenges the commonly held notion that women in the life are sick and weak (Sabella Monheit, 2010):

> Marie rejects the notion, as did a number of other women in the study, that women in prostitution are sick and weak and makes the point that they should not be typecast as such, especially when one considers what women like her have experienced and survived. Although she acknowledges women in prostitution certainly have their issues, she believes they have their strengths as well. In her statement that follows, she emphasizes the word "not," making it clear that she never saw herself as a victim and does not want others to view her or other women involved in prostitution as such either. It was important to her that she and other women be recognized more for their strength and for being strong, and for the many positive things they have to offer:
>
> > I get really angry when people make us sicker than we really are. Don't make us sicker than we really are. Listen, you can survive a day on the street, you can survive most anything. Do not be thinking that they [the women] can't talk about things or they can't do certain things. Some need more help than others, they really do, but we are not victims. People who survive the streets are strong. So don't underestimate them. We're strong powerful women with a lot of things to offer. (p. 268)
>
> Marie continues to share her view of herself, focusing on how she saw herself as a prostitute. Marie, by her own words "not the best prostitute," also spoke of her prostitution identity having to be fake and how it was difficult to reconcile that with her sense of who Marie was, an honest person. No one had the option to be who she really was in the life as who would pay to have sex with someone who hated sex, had a headache, or who just wanted to get the money as quickly as possible so she could make a car payment before the car got repossessed. For Marie, her prostitution identity was all fake and a lie, having nothing to do with who she was or wanted to be. To fake it meant having to put on a happy face as the show must go on:
>
> > In the beginning, you have this sense that you're somebody out there. And what happens is, um, you start to realize that you're

really nobody. You have to keep a façade up because you don't make money if you show the real side of yourself. Nobody's paying you to get in a car and say, Jesus, I'm having a lousy day. Like, will you listen to my problems? Nobody wants to hear when they pay you for a blow job that you don't like doing blow jobs—and that you're doing it because you don't—you feel like you've run out—you have no other choice. So, it all becomes a lie and, and, and unless you're really delusional, you know that. You know that. But you may not outwardly show that to the world. I'll fake it if I have to. You have to do that to make the money, but that was really hard for me. Being a phony, like that was really hard for me. (p. 287)

In this chapter I also shared the themes related to relationships and belonging, and how, for some women, being in the life provided them with a sense of belonging. This excerpt focuses on relationships of belonging and details how prostitution served that purpose for Crystal (Sabella Monheit, 2010):

While being involved with men was important, not all the women's desires for relationships centered on men, romance, or material gain. What many of the women wanted and sought was a relationship with no sex attached, a relationship that could serve as a substitute for family or a relationship with a group they felt comfortable with. For a number of the women, being involved in prostitution gave them a sense of belonging, something that they had not experienced much of before in their lives, and being in the life allowed them to reach out and touch others who were at the same place and space as they were. Being involved in prostitution allowed them to forge relationships with others whom they felt were "their people," those also involved in the life. As mentioned at the beginning of this chapter, Gee (2000) speaks of an affinity identity. As the women accepted that identity, of being connected and affiliated with others in the life, they also connected through forming actual relationships with women also in the life. Here Crystal describes part of what kept her out there, which was the importance she attached to her relationship of finally belonging to the right club. Her sense of belonging was founded on the fact that she shared a similar background and experiences with "her people" and that they all shared similar activities. In short, they were all from the same country and spoke the same language. We know it is human nature to want to belong and to seek out those like ourselves. Through prostitution Crystal has finally found a place to call home among the people she can call her people:

I never knew that there was anything outside of prostitution and drugs. I never knew that I could be cared for and loved without giving my all or money to someone. I also liked the sense of belonging, cause I knew who my people were, where I belonged, who I belonged to. I can't connect with the educated people 'cause I'm not educated. I can't connect with the well-off, well-to-do people 'cause, you know, when I was hungry, when I was growing up I ate dirt, you know because we didn't have food all the time. We didn't have meat all the time. You know, so I can't— I'm just like totally ghetto-fied, but I'm not as ghetto as the ghetto. So I, you know, I—the only place I fit in was way down, down at the bottom of the food chain. It was camaraderie, you know what I mean? Because we was all out there doing the same thing. I knew I belonged to that group of ghetto hustlers. (pp. 325–326)

Dissemination

As of this writing, I have not done much to disseminate my work in large measure. The dissertation was submitted to ProQuest LLC and is available in the University of Pennsylvania library. I have shared my work and findings in several presentations I have given related to prostitution and human trafficking, and I have personally used the findings in my work in various therapy groups I conduct for women involved in prostitution. In addition, in some of my publications, I reference my dissertation and findings, and I post some of my chapters for students to read in a course I teach on human trafficking. Although I have no doubt that the work would be of interest and value to a larger audience, I found that after completion of the dissertation I did not devote myself to making as much effort as I should have to publishing. Instead, I found and still find myself working on other publications that include articles and chapters in a number of other areas aside from prostitution. I am also a managing editor for a mental health column in the *American Journal of Nursing* and was recently appointed managing editor for a journal on human trafficking which is slated to begin publication in 2015. Those duties and my full-time position in an academic setting do not leave much time for working on disseminating my dissertation work.

SUMMARY

All told, this was an amazing journey. I was blessed by having a chair who was open to accompanying me, sometimes to places that were probably new to her, and who gave graciously of her time and knowledge. I also had a committee who were level-headed, supportive, and understood what I was trying to do. They gave good advice and did not get caught up in minutia and trivia. I am forever grateful to each one of them for not making my life a living hell, as I heard horror stories from colleagues for whom that had been the case in their own experiences at other institutions. In my opinion, choosing your committee as wisely as you can and as freely as you have the power to do so is extremely important. My next piece of advice is to choose a topic that really means something to you and about which you feel some excitement and interest, and, perhaps if you're lucky like me, about which you feel some passion. There are an awful lot of words that go into writing a dissertation and if you find yourself turned off and just going through the motions early on, each word will only add to that burden in ways that give new meaning to the term "torture." I felt a burning desire to understand what life in prostitution was like for the women I interviewed, and even perhaps more importantly and on a grander level, I felt a connection to them as universal sisters. Because of the public stigma that often colors their existence and silences their voices, I wanted to offer my voice through which they could tell their stories. For me this was not just an act of labor, but a labor of love. I realize that not everyone reading this is a mental health nurse who has the opportunity or desire to connect with their participants in a manner or level similar to what I did, which is fine, as we all approach our research and dissertation from different contexts and perspectives. But nonetheless, the more you are interested and excited by what you're about to do, the more likely it is that you will enjoy the process.

Aside from the advantages mentioned in the preceding paragraph, once I stopped fooling around and tricking myself into thinking that I needed to read one more article to discover some great mystery, I found it helpful to set up a writing schedule and stick with it. No dissertation that is unattended or ignored will write itself. The dissertation will depend entirely on you to take it to completion, so do set up a schedule that is reasonable for your life, but consistent, and make it a point to work on it as often as possible. It's worth the sacrifice of missing out on some things to get this done sooner rather than later.

And finally, enjoy the ride. Doing research will take you places you may never have imagined and could allow you access to information and experiences you may never have had or will have again. Each time I sat with a woman for our interview I felt like it was Christmas and her story was the gift she was giving me. Once we started our interview, I began to unwrap this wonderful present with no idea what was inside and what was to come. This was not something I did every day, but as a researcher, I was now granted permission to be transported to places I wanted to go to but could not get to on my own. Yes, I was doing this because it was the final requirement to obtain the coveted degree, but eventually it went beyond that to my doing it to gain the information and understanding to become a better therapist and mental health nurse for the women with whom I was and would be working. Indeed, there were times when I was frustrated and tired and asked myself why I was doing this, but I tried to never lose sight of the light at the end of the tunnel. I am grateful for the experience and wish you the best as you begin yours. If you are curious about a given phenomenon and want the opportunity to find out more about it on a level deeper and richer than possible with some other methods, I highly recommend that you consider taking a phenomenological approach. For me, doing so was the right ticket to get me where I wanted to go!

REFERENCES

Arrington, M. (1987). *Good girls, bad girls: Sex trade workers and feminists face to face.* London, UK: The Women's Press.

Baker, L., Case, P., & Policicchio, D. (2005). General health problems of inner-city sex workers: A pilot study. *Journal of Medical Library Association, 9*(1), 67–71.

Baker, L., Wilson, F., & Wineberger, A. (2004). An exploratory study of the health problems, stigmatization, life satisfaction and literacy skills of urban street-level sex workers. *Women and Health, 39*(2), 83–96.

Basserman, L. (1993). *The oldest profession: A history of prostitution.* New York, NY: Hermann Schreiber.

Baumgartner, L. (2000). *Narrative analysis: Uncovering the truth of stories.* Retrieved September 3, 2008 from http://www.edst.educ.ubc.ca/aerc/2000/baumgartnerl1-final.pdf

Boyd, C. O. (2001). Phenomenology: The method. In P. L. Munhall (Ed.), *Nursing research: A qualitative perspective* (3rd ed., pp. 93–122). Sudbury, MA: Jones and Bartlett.

Boynton, P. (2002). Life on the streets: The experiences of community researchers in a study of prostitution. *Journal of Community and Applied Social Psychology, 12*(1), 1–12.

Braun, V., & Clarke, V. (2006). Using thematic analysis in psychology. *Qualitative Research in Psychology, 3,* 77–101.

Chancer, L. (1993). Prostitution, feminist theory and ambivalence: Notes from the sociological underground. *Social Text, 37,* 143–171.

Charon, R. (2007). What to do with stories: The sciences of narrative medicine. *Canadian Family Physician, 53*(8), 1265–1267.

Creswell, J. W. (1998). *Qualitative inquiry and research design: Choosing among five traditions.* Thousand Oaks, CA: Sage Publications.

Daiute, C., & Lightfoot, C. (Eds.). (2004). *Narrative analysis: Studying the development of individuals in society.* London, UK: Sage Publications.

Dalla, R. L. (2006a). *Exposing the pretty woman myth: A qualitative investigation of street-level prostituted women.* Lanham, MD: Lexington Books.

Davidson, L. (2003). *Living outside mental illness: Qualitative studies of recovery in schizophrenia.* New York, NY: New York University Press.

Denzin, N. K. (1989). *Interpretive biography.* London, UK: Sage Publications.

Dickens, C. (1859). *A tale of two cities.* London, UK: Chapman and Hall.

Elliott, J. (2005). *Using narrative in social research: Qualitative and quantitative approaches.* London, UK: Sage Publications.

Evans, H. (1979). *Harlots, whores and hookers: A history of prostitution.* New York, NY: Taplinger Publishing.

Farley, M. (2003a). Prostitution and the invisibility of harm. *Women and Therapy, 26*(3,4), 247–280.

Farley, M. (Ed.). (2003b). *Prostitution, trafficking and traumatic stress.* Binghamton, NY: The Haworth Maltreatment & Trauma Press.

Farley, M., & Kelly, V. (2000). Prostitution: A critical review of the medical and social sciences literature. *Women and Critical Justice, 11*(4), 29–64.

Gee, J. P. (2000). Chapter 3: Identity as an analytic lens for research in education. *Review of Research in Education, 25,* 99–125.

Goffman, E. (1963). *Stigma: Notes on the management of spoiled identity.* New York, NY: Simon & Schuster.

Groenewald, T. (2004). A phenomenological research design illustrated. *International Journal of Qualitative Methods, 3*(1), 1–26.

Hedin, U., & Mansson, S. (2003). The importance of supportive relationships among women leaving prostitution. *Journal of Trauma Practice, 2*(3/4), 223–237.

Hester, M., & Westmarland, N. (2004). Tackling street prostitution: Towards an holistic approach. London: Home Office Research Studies. Retrieved June 7, 2006, from http://www.homeoffice.gov.uk/rds/index.htm

Hiles, D. (2007). Identity positioning: Narrative analysis of Sjuzet and Fabula. *Narrative and Memory.* Retrieved September 1, 2009, from http://www.2.hud.ac.uk/hhs.nme/bppks/2007/Chapter_4_-David_Hiles.pdf

Hycner, R. H. (1999). Some guidelines for the phenomenological analysis of interview data. In A. Bryman & R. G. Burgess (Eds.), *Qualitative research 3* (pp. 143, 164). London, UK: Sage Publications.

Jeal, N., & Salisbury, C. (2004). A health needs assessment of street-based prostitutes: Cross-sectional survey. *Journal of Public Health, 26*(2), 147–151.

Jolin, A. (1994). On the backs of the working prostitutes: Feminist theory and prostitution policy. *Crime and Delinquency, 40*(1), 69–83.

Labov, W., & Waletzky, J. (1967). Narrative analysis: Oral versions of personal experience. In J. Helm (Ed.), *Essays on the verbal and visual arts* (pp. 12–44). Seattle, WA: University of Washington Press.

Labov, W., & Waletzky, J. (1997). Narrative analysis: Oral versions of personal experience. *Journal of Narrative and Life History, 7*(1–4), 3–38. Retrieved September 15, 2008, from http://www.clarku.edu/-mbamberg/LabovWaletzky.htm

Liamputtong, P. (2007). *Researching the vulnerable: A guide to sensitive research methods.* Thousand Oaks, CA: Sage Publications.

Lieblich, A., Tuval-Mashiach, R., & Zilber, T. (1998). *Narrative research: Reading, analysis and interpretation*. Thousand Oaks, CA: Sage Publications.

Lysaker, P., & Buck, K. (2006). Moving toward recovery within clients' personal narratives: Directions for a recovery-focused therapy. *Journal of Psychosocial Nursing & Mental Health Services, 44*(1), 29–35.

Maxwell, J. A. (2005). *Qualitative research design: An interactive approach* (2nd ed.). Thousand Oaks, CA: Sage Publications.

McAdams, D. (1993). *The stories we live by: Personal myths and the making of the self*. New York, NY: Morrow.

McLeod, J. (2001). *Qualitative research in counseling and psychotherapy*. London, UK: Sage Publications.

Melrose, M. (2002). Labour pains: Some considerations on the difficulties of researching juvenile prostitution. *International Journal of Social Research Methodology, 5*(4), 333–351.

Mishler, E. G. (1986a). The analysis of interview narratives. In T. R. Sarbin (Ed.), *Narrative psychology: The storied nature of human conduct* (pp. 233–255). New York, NY: Praeger.

Mishler, E. G. (1986b). *Research interviewing: Context and narrative*. Cambridge, MA: Harvard University Press.

Mishler, E. G. (1995). Models of narrative analysis: A typology. *Journal of Narrative and Life History, 5*(2), 87–123.

Murray, M. (2000). Levels of narrative analysis in health psychology. *Journal of Health Psychology, 5*(3), 337–347.

Napoli, M., Gerdes, K., & DeSouza-Rowland, S. (2001). Treatment of prostitution using integrative therapy techniques: A case study. *Journal of Contemporary Psychotherapy, 31*(2), 71–87.

Oakley, A. (Ed.). (2007). *Working sex: Sex workers write about a changing industry*. Emeryville, CA: Seal Press.

Parker, J. (1998). *How prostitution works*. Retrieved June 11, 2006, from www.prostitutionresearch.com

Phoenix, J. (1999). *Making sense of prostitution*. Basingstoke, UK: Macmillan.

Phoenix, J. (2000). Prostitute identities. *The British Journal of Criminology 40*(1), 37–55.

Riessman, C. K. (1993). *Narrative analysis*. London, UK: Sage Publications.

Riessman, C. K. (2008). *Narrative methods for the human sciences*. Thousand Oaks, CA: Sage Publications.

Ringdal, N. J. (2004*). Love for sale: A world history of prostitution*. New York, NY: Grove Press.

Roberts, N. (1986). *The front line: Women in the sex industry speak*. London, UK: Grafton.

Roberts, N. (1992). *Whores in history: Prostitution in western society*. London, UK: HarperCollins Publishers.

Rymes, B. (2001). *Conversational borderlands: Language and identity in an alternative urban high school*. New York, NY: Teachers College Press.

Sabella Monheit, D. (2010). *Lives in the life: Making sense of prostitution through narrative*. (Doctoral dissertation). Philadelphia, PA: University of Pennsylvania. Retrieved from http://repository.upenn.edu/dissertations/AAI3447144/

Scoular, J. (2004). The "subject" of prostitution: Interpreting the discursive, symbolic and material position of sex/work in feminist theory. *Feminist Theory, 5*(3), 343–355.

Seidman, I. (1998). *Interviewing as qualitative research.* New York, NY: Teacher's College Press.

Shaver, F. (2005). Sex work research: Methodological and ethical challenges. *Journal of Interpersonal Violence, 20*(3), 296–319.

Tomura, M. (2009). A prostitute's lived experience of stigma. *Journal of Phenomenological Psychology, 40*(1), 51–84.

Valera, R., Sawyer, R., & Schiraldi, G. (2001). Perceived health needs of inner-city street prostitutes: A preliminary study. *American Journal of Health Behavior, 25*(1), 50–59.

van Manen, M. (1990). *Researching lived experience: Human science for an action sensitive pedagogy.* Albany, NY: State University of New York Press.

Weiner, A. (1996). Understanding the social needs of streetwalking prostitutes. *Social Work, 41*(1), 97–105.

Williamson, C., & Folaron, G. (2001). Violence, risk and survival strategies of street prostitution. *Western Journal of Nursing Research, 23*, 463–475.

Williamson, C., & Folaron, G. (2003). Understanding the experiences of street level prostitutes. *Qualitative Social Work, 2*(3), 271–287.

Young, A., Boyd, C., & Hubbell, A. (2000). Prostitution, drug use, and coping with psychological distress. *Journal of Drug Issues, 30*(4), 789–800.

Zweig, J., Schlichter, K., & Burt, M. (2002). Assisting women victims of violence who experience multiple barriers to services. *Violence Against Women, 8*(2), 162–180.

CHAPTER FIVE

KISSING FROGS: FINDING THE RIGHT PHENOMENOLOGIST FOR FRAMING QUALITATIVE INQUIRY IN NURSING

Rebecca Green

What is this stupid frog trying to say? He just sits here in the water with his own kind and croaks. He cannot be a companion to a human.

(Grimm & Grimm, 1812)

The reason why the idiom "you have to kiss a lot of frogs before you find a prince" is so enduring is because it resonates for many people who weather a lot of less-than-satisfactory relationships before finding the perfect partner who fulfills every need and desire. But what of the poor frogs, reviled over and over by fair and facile maidens looking for the perfect mate? The Scottish origin of this well-used turn of phrase reveals a far more complex story than popular understanding suggests: One maiden's frog is another's prince (Campbell, 1969); or, any frog could be a prince for the right person under the right circumstances, given an opportunity and a little commitment (Grimm & Grimm, 1812).

Let me assure readers, who may be wondering exactly what kissing frogs has to do with nursing research and phenomenology, that the experience of finding just the right phenomenologist to illuminate the conceptual intricacies of a novice researcher's topic of study is not at all dissimilar from kissing many, many, cool, moist, and rough-textured amphibians, each time in the hope that it will transform into, if not a stalwart prince on a white steed, then a phenomenologist whose particular way of characterizing the discipline, the study, and the methods of phenomenology will be "the right one" for that researcher and for that study.

THE NOVICE RESEARCHER

I mentioned that I was a novice researcher. Indeed, I was about as new to independent research as a person can be. Over the course of two semesters, in the latter half of my doctoral program, I took courses both in qualitative inquiry and a practicum in applied nursing research. I drew on my interest, some previous projects, and some reading, and developed a concrete project that included a pilot interview questionnaire and the institutional review board (IRB) proposal and approval. The course in qualitative inquiry is what made me certain that I had found my home as a researcher. Although I like quantitative inquiry, and, in fact, decided to pursue doctoral studies because of a desire to strengthen my skills in quantitative research, the course in qualitative inquiry had me more interested in research than I had ever been before. The research practicum allowed me to expand a project I had started in the qualitative inquiry course. One of the most important exercises in the practicum was the maintenance of a project journal in which, as students, we were required to keep a detailed record of our activities related to the research we were doing, the communications we had on the research, and the reflective processes we engaged in as we went through the process. This journaling was time consuming, but it provided a valuable record of the entire research process and the minute details that would otherwise have been forgotten. Many articles and texts on any type of research urge investigators to keep a detailed record of each step of the investigative process (National Institutes of Health, 2008; Ortlipp, 2008), much like the journal activity I described earlier, but I wonder how often this practice is faithfully observed. I am grateful to the professor in that course who introduced it to us early and encouraged us to make a careful habit of it. This work in this course, after a lot of blood, sweat, and tears, eventually became my dissertation proposal during my dissertation seminar in the summer of 2011. The study I describe in this chapter is my dissertation research, and much of the content herein comes directly and verbatim from my dissertation (Green, 2012).

It is important for the reader to understand a little about what generated my interest in my dissertation topic. I am a White woman, born in Atlanta at the height of the civil rights movement and raised in the southern United States. I have been intrigued by the intricacies of interpersonal race relationships as long as I can remember, probably beginning at about age 8, when I asked my mother, who led my Girl Scout group in the very White Atlanta suburbs in the 1970s, why she drove downtown every Tuesday afternoon to do the exact same thing in Capitol Homes, an urban housing project, with a group of little Black girls—earning badges, making crafts, singing songs, planning camp-outs. I remember being perplexed by her response, which involved becoming teary and telling me that it was "important." That was the extent of it and, ever since, I have been looking for a better explanation.

My first job as a nurse, more than 20 years ago, was working in Oakland, California, in a neonatal intensive care unit, and my most recent job in the clinical setting was as a school nurse in an inner-city middle school in south Georgia. My experiences in every health care setting have led to my observation that health care encounters are often fraught with social, economic, gender, and professional inequity; an inequity that may establish professional bias and lead to unquestioned assumptions about which the professional practitioner may not be aware in daily interactions and encounters with patients (Green, 2012). In my practice as a pediatric nurse, I was especially concerned about clinician relationships with African American parents and how those relationships affected the health of the child. My own personal history and practice experiences drove my scholarly inquiry.

I was interested in gaining a deeper, richer understanding of what occurred during encounters and in gaining insight into personal, familial, and sociocultural forces that shaped the encounters from the point of view of parents (Green, 2012). So how did I come to choose a qualitative design to gain this insight and generate this understanding? The very definition of qualitative inquiry will enlighten the reader as to why the only logical choice for this line of inquiry was a qualitative design, because "qualitative research is known for giving voice to people, to hearing people's own personal narrative, and using the language of our participants to research" (Munhall, 2007, p. 4). I was interested in gaining an understanding about the social worlds of parents and children, about how their social lives influenced their experiences and interactions with providers, and how they interpreted their experiences. These are points of understanding that would distinguish a dynamic, qualitative approach to inquiry (Beneloiel, 1984). Another motivational factor in the choice of a qualitative design was the question of whether a White scholar could engage in legitimate research about race and ethnicity of African Americans. Tillman (2002) addressed this question by recommending that such research can be done if the researcher eschews a deficit view of the culture being studied and has a relationship with the community; if the method used is qualitative; if the data interpretation is culturally sensitive; and if the research seeks culturally specific knowledge, reveals unequal power relations, and leads to the development of culture-specific theory and interventions (Tillman, 2002).

As I designed the study, I kept Tillman's (2002) tenets in mind, one of which, of course, is that the design be qualitative. But beyond qualitative design, which methodology was most appropriate? This was a particularly difficult puzzle for me to solve as a novice researcher. As I developed the proposal and refined the specific research questions, I continued to struggle with elements of various methodologies, as do many novice researchers: What, exactly, was I doing? I had designed my study as a critical ethnography. But what was the appropriate phenomenological framework? I am a person who loves order! I needed clarity. My dissertation chair, a Heideggerian phenomenologist, kept reminding me that much qualitative inquiry is rooted in phenomenology, an idea echoed by Munhall (2007) and by Guest, Namey, and Mitchell (2013). She also kept reminding me that qualitative inquiry is often messy. I felt I needed to immerse myself in phenomenology, and better grasp salient differences among different phenomenological approaches, before I made a decision about a phenomenological lens. And so the summer of kissing frogs commenced.

At the time I was enrolled in my doctoral program, I had the good fortune to be employed as a school nurse, so I had two long months of summer stretching out ahead of me, during which I was determined to become more broadly read in phenomenology. I have the marvelous fortune to be married to a professor of religious studies, whose extensive library (and philosophical expertise) was at my ready disposal (and I did a lot of disposing)! I had done a great deal of preplanning and research and had selected several potential phenomenological approaches that might provide the perfect philosophical foundation for framing my inquiry. Who were the lucky suitors? Husserl, Heidegger, Sartre, Ricoeur, Merleau-Ponty, and Edith Stein. As I embarked on my journey with each of these phenomenologists, I felt cautious excitement. I will not spend a great deal of time discussing the distinct perspectives of each of these phenomenologists, as this is not the purpose of my work here, nor would it be remotely possible in a single chapter to do justice to even one. Although reading their work certainly broadened my understanding and strengthened my grasp of phenomenology, certainly enough for writing the necessary dissertation chapter justifying a qualitative, phenomenological approach to my inquiry, not one of these really spoke to me as being the perfect fit for really illuminating my work uniquely.

When I finally got to Merleau-Ponty, like the last match in a round of speed dating, I had really high hopes. As I look back now at my well-thumbed and highlighted copy of Patricia Munhall's *Qualitative Inquiry in Nursing*, I even see that I had underlined the following sentence: "Merleau-Ponty's work is particularly important to the health sciences because of his investigations on the role of the body in perception and society" (Dombro, 2007, p. 116). I desperately wanted this one to work out, but alas, another instance of an interesting fellow, but no real chemistry. Maybe I was taking the wrong approach altogether. Who needs a man anyway? Well, a fish may not need a bicycle (Martin, 2013), but I still needed a phenomenologist; thus, I turned to a woman to seek some enlightenment. Edith Stein was a student of Husserl and a very productive scholar and writer. Her early work centered on the concept of empathy (Stein & Stein, 1989). Her mature work, however, although appropriate and applicable to the questions I was asking, were of a decidedly religious nature (she had converted to Catholicism and entered a Carmelite monastery) (International Association for the Study of the Philosophy of Edith Stein [IASPES], 2009).

In each case, my hopes were dashed. Another poor fit. I felt frustrated, confused, and honestly tired of kissing frogs. And this was challenging reading! I kept hearkening back to my first doctoral course, philosophy of science, when many of us were lamenting how very difficult the readings were, how challenging the concepts were to grasp. The lamentations had gone on for some time when one of the professors who cotaught the course finally had had enough and said to us, "You have *got* to stop saying that. It is a self-fulfilling prophecy. Of course you won't understand it if you tell yourselves and each other that you can't understand it. You are intelligent women, perfectly capable of understanding and grasping this material. Of course it is hard. This is a doctoral program." As I read through the works of my selected suitors, these words echoed resoundingly in my head. Yes, that professor was, in fact, my dissertation chair! Perhaps I should just give up. There was no phenomenologist for me. No perfect one. Or maybe I should not give up, but just make do with one I had already kissed, accepting life with a frog on the pillow next to me, instead of seeking some nonexistent ideal.

Then my fairy godmother (my husband, I mean) recommended that I dip my toes in just one more proverbial pond. And here let me interject a word to the wise: Take help and advice graciously whenever it is offered and from whomever it comes. For quite some time, I had resisted asking my husband's opinion about phenomenology, because I wanted to be completely independent in this process. When he recommended that I consider reading the work of Alfred Schutz, my response was, "But you are an expert on Alfred Schutz." He said, "That is why I am so certain that his work will fit the questions you are concerned about. Please, just read his work, and see what I mean." After I read Schutz's collected papers (1962, 1964), there was no question in my mind that I had finally kissed the right frog. I kissed my husband, too! Interestingly, Schutz's work was no less difficult, no less complex than that of any of the other phenomenologists I had read thus far. But his work resonated with me. It felt right. It fit. Having to read and reread passages did not make me frustrated: Instead, doing so excited me as

I gained better understanding, as I realized just how perfectly Schutz's social phenomenology framed the questions to which I was seeking answers and created an obvious avenue for the seamless integration of elements of the other theory and method (narrative and critical ethnography) into what was essentially a phenomenological inquiry.

But I still felt funny about choosing Schutz and living in the house with a scholar of Schutz. I called my dissertation chair to discuss what I thought could be a problem. I did not want anyone to think that my husband in any way "helped" me write my dissertation. Her response was, "Consider yourself lucky. Not everyone has a resident philosopher in the house when they are writing a dissertation. He can be helpful to you without helping you write your dissertation." This is how I came to choose the social phenomenology of Alfred Schutz as an interpretive framework that allowed me to blend essential elements of phenomenology, critical ethnography, and narrative inquiry into my dissertation: *African American Parents' Experiences in their Children's Health Care Encounters.*

When I had read Schutz's work, it became clear that it made sense to use social phenomenology as the interpretive lens for my particular study. Many novice researchers are confused, as I was, by the overlapping and fuzzy boundaries of the various qualitative methodologies. For a while, I was convinced that my study was narrative, because I was interested in the stories parents had to tell about their encounters. And this is true! Creswell (2007, p. 54) discussed narrative as both a methodology and a phenomenon of study, and as a term that could be "assigned to any text or discourse." But then I came to realize that while I was indeed interested in stories, I was interested in more than the series of actions or chronology of life events, which generally characterize narratives (Czarniawska, 2004).

Yes, I was interested in the narratives African American parents had to tell about encounters they had with their children in health care settings. But this was in no way a simple ethnography, because I did not wish to record the pattern of behavior, language, and belief of African Americans in the anthropological sense. I was really more interested in the intersection of two cultures: a minority culture and the dominant health care culture. Thinking back to Tillman's requirement for majority researchers to pay careful attention to power imbalances and inequity in relationships, I knew I wanted these to be central to my consideration, and so it seemed appropriate to consider that my inquiry would at least incorporate elements of critical ethnography. Critical ethnography is research through which authors seek to expose power, prestige, privilege, and authority used to oppress minority groups and advocate for the emancipation of those marginalized groups

(Creswell, 2007; Thomas, 1993). So yes, I *was* doing critical ethnography, and yes, I was evaluating narratives. This intentional blending of methodologies has been referred to as *bricolage* (Kincheloe & Berry, 2004). Let me explain how beautifully Alfred Schutz allowed me to include elements of all of these under the umbrella of social phenomenology.

Chapter 3 of my dissertation was titled *Philosophy, Methodology and Theoretical Frameworks*. It is important to recognize that while rigid adherence to a particular methodology is not necessary and is actually antithetical to the qualitative approach (Janesick, 1994; Sandelowski, 1993; Thorne, 2011), the qualitative researcher is not free to be *amethodological* or without understanding of method or the theory behind method. In fact, the more comprehensive a researcher's understanding of a variety of methodological and theoretical approaches, the greater the research potential. Thorne (2011) said it well: "A health science researcher overly attached to any one theoretical perspective is understood ... to have lost his or her ontological moorings" (p. 448). While I do not claim to be an expert in method, methodology, or theory, I do claim to have made an exhaustive effort in terms of preparing myself and understanding all three in order to approach my topic in a reasoned and reasonable manner.

Chapter 3 (Green, 2012) represented my effort to link the conceptual and theoretical tenets of the philosophy undergirding the qualitative approach, the social phenomenology of Alfred Schutz as an interpretive phenomenological paradigm, and the methodology and theory underlying critical ethnography to justify my approach to and the design of the proposed study. I demonstrated how they are theoretically related, how they informed one another, and how they grounded my inquiry into African American parents' experiences of their children's health care encounters. The most important realization about phenomenology, said Munhall (2007, p. 148), is that "two different perceptions are going to result in two different interpretations of what seemingly looks like one reality." It is this realization that propels qualitative inquiry.

Alfred Schutz was a phenomenologist who broadened the scope of individual phenomenology to encompass the social world (Barber, 2011). Schutz was born in Vienna at the turn of the 20th century and, as a young man, studied law, social science, and economics. He was strongly influenced by the writing of Max Weber, a sociologist, and Edmund Husserl, who is considered by many to be the founder of contemporary phenomenology (Barber, 2011). Schutz placed emphasis on personal action and motive, and understanding of other's actions and motives, which moves phenomenology beyond perceived experience into the realm of moral action.

Alfred Schutz (1962, p. 9) placed daily human social interaction within a context of "biographically determined situations" which are defined by the individual and dependent on that individual's unique physical space, time, status, role, and ideological position. Some of these elements are imposed, whereas others are within the realm of individual control. Schutz (1962, p. 10) referred to our human existence together as "an intersubjective world of culture" in which we are bound by common influence and mutual understanding manifest in "textures of meaning." Textures of meaning originate in human action in the form of *historicity*, our own and our predecessors' tools, language, art, and social institutions. Schutz (1962, p. 10) described historicity (tradition and culture) as the sediment of human activity. Intersubjectivity is the capacity of human consciousness to be aware of realities that are not directly available to the self but that are being experienced by others, the awareness of and sharing the experience of others through the medium of human communication (Stoltzfus, 1998). Language and vocabulary are two of the primary mediums through which historicity is transmitted, in what Schutz (1962, p. 14) refers to as the "vernacular of everyday life"; therefore, the media of language and vocabulary were central to my choice of face-to-face interviews as method.

Schutz was also interested in the concepts of equality and deliberative democracy (Barber, 2011). Given Schutz's concepts of intersubjective participation, culture, historicity, and equality, it is no surprise that his social phenomenology is widely used by critical ethnographers. Philosophical concepts similar to Schutz's are reflected in the methodology of critical ethnography and in its foundational theoretical framework, critical social theory. Schutz's (1962, p. 10) characterization of human interaction as "an intersubjective world of culture" and the tenets of his social phenomenology are particularly appropriate as a foundation for critical ethnographic inquiry.

Critical ethnography originated in the discipline of anthropology and assumes social justice, critical theory, and phenomenological perspectives to illuminate social action. Madison described critical ethnography as "critical theory in action" (2005, p. 13). Thomas (1993, p. 5) described ethnographic emancipation as "the act of cultural liberation, [which] loosens the unrecognized symbolic constraints that restrict our perception, interpretation, discourse, and action" and defines critical ethnography as

> a type of reflection that examines culture, knowledge, and action. It expands our horizons for choice and widens our experiential capacity to see, hear, and feel. It deepens and sharpens ethical commitments by forcing us to develop and act upon value commitments in the context

of political agendas. Critical ethnographers describe, analyze, and open to scrutiny otherwise hidden agendas, power centers, and assumptions that inhibit, repress, and constrain. (Thomas, 1993, p. 2)

Critical ethnography differs from standard ethnography in that it is openly value-laden and its purpose is emancipation: emancipation of all those within the marginalizing relationship or system (not only the marginalized but also the unmarginalized, dominant groups). Usually a critical ethnographer identifies an overriding theme of interest—for example, the health of African American children—and seeks to analyze how the cultural group of interest is influenced by power and inequity in the greater cultural milieu. The purpose of my study was to investigate the experiences that African American parents have in their children's health care encounters. My assumption, from a critical perspective, was that inequities exist in the health care system and that power imbalances exist within health care relationships. It was through a critical lens that I viewed the data I gathered from interviews with African American parents. A variety of components, such as history, politics, economy, and environment, were considered when identifying characteristics of and influences on the cultural groups: African American parents and health care providers. Schutz would call these components part of the biological situation and historicity. I had particular interest in how African American parents experienced their children's health care encounters. It was not only their perceptions of the encounters that were significant, but also the conventions, values, and beliefs about health care and institutional professionals that precede and define the encounters— what Duffy (2007, p. 402) called "interface" of the African American parents' "personal and social identity with the social world" in the context of health care encounters and interaction with health care professionals.

Qualitative inquiry honors the subjective nature of reality, and the many meanings that may be inherent in a particular phenomenon or experience. The social phenomenology of Alfred Schutz, with its focus on the intersubjectivity of the social world, provided an interpretive framework for considering the experiences of African American parents in their children's health care encounters. Critical ethnography, with the dual components of ethnographic and critical analysis, was a useful methodological tool for analyzing these experiences within the Schutzian framework and helping me focus on an overall aim in my study: to gain an understanding of the personal, familial, and sociocultural forces that shape African American parents' encounters with health care providers and the health care system. But analysis can only occur when one has a body of data to analyze, and a great deal of work went into designing and operationalizing this study.

THE NUTS AND BOLTS

In this second half of this chapter, I will discuss the nuts and bolts of the study—the sample, the setting, IRB, instrumentation, data collection, and timeline—so the reader can see how conceptual and practical difficulties were resolved and the design became operational. The majority of the second half of the chapter will be spent on a discussion of the analysis of data after they were generated within the Schutzian framework. It was a fascinating process, and novice researchers may gain insight into the process from reading about my own experience.

I mentioned earlier my doctoral course in qualitative inquiry and research practicum where I drew on my interest, some previous projects, and some reading and developed a concrete project that included a pilot interview questionnaire and the IRB proposal and approval. The primary data collection method I employed was face-to-face, open-ended, semi-structured interviews with African American parents, which were digitally recorded and transcribed verbatim. There were several background and demographic questions, which included questions about age, family description, income level, and employment. The preliminary guide consisted of a series of about 20 questions I developed from reading Madison's (2005) text on critical ethnography in which she evaluated several models for interviewing. The Spradley model categorized questions, in part, as "tour questions," which address concrete situational descriptions of phenomena; "example questions," which ask the participant to recount an experience that best exemplifies the experience of a phenomenon; and "experience questions," which ask the participant to detail the experience of a particular phenomenon (Madison, 2005, p. 28). These characterizations of questions helped me develop the questions that I would use to loosely guide each interview.

Once I had developed a general direction of inquiry, purpose, and interview guide, I proposed the study to the university's IRB, and it was quickly approved in January 2011. I proposed a pilot study, using seven participants, to refine the guide I used in the larger study, based on input from the participants. The pilot study was critical to the development of a usable instrument and for the purpose of developing my comfort and skill as a novice interviewer. Flexibility in the semistructured interview is what I had been hoping to gain during the pilot process. In the qualitative interview, over adherence to a guide can inhibit the process and preclude the possibility of discovering "how the interviewee frames and understands issues and events—that is, what the interviewee views as important in explaining and understanding events, patterns, and forms of behavior" (Bryman, 2004, p. 314). Several months later, the IRB approved the continuation of the study using the revised guide, which, in fact, had had some elements removed.

Various methods of purposive sampling were employed to recruit African American parents aged 18 to 60 from a variety of backgrounds and occupations throughout south Georgia. Participants were identified through professional and personal contacts through a school system. The first seven participants were those who participated in the pilot study. They were contacts and acquaintances I had from my work as a school nurse. Four additional participants were recruited through letters sent home to students of one small elementary school (with permission from the superintendent and board of education). School nurses in the local city school system, with the permission of the superintendent, asked parents with whom they had contact by telephone or face-to-face contact over a period of one week if they would like to participate in a voluntary research project. If they indicated interest, they were given my phone number; thus, five more participants were recruited. Chain referral (snowballing) by participants resulted, during the research process, in identifying two additional eligible participants, who were given my contact information by other participants. Interviews of the 18 participants were conducted in places the participants chose, with attention to ensure enough privacy to guarantee confidentiality. Interview locations on most occasions were participants' homes; but I also interviewed them in my home, in a secluded booth in a fast-food restaurant, at a local park with playground equipment to occupy the participant's energetic children, in the school clinic where I work and see children (after hours), and at a school library at the school where a participant worked.

Data collection, in the form of interviewing, commenced in February of 2011, as soon as I received IRB approval for the pilot study, and continued through mid-summer of the same year after I received IRB approval for an expansion of the study for my dissertation. Interviews were transcribed verbatim. I transcribed the first seven, and had the last eleven transcribed professionally so that I could focus on data analysis. I did preliminary identification of significant statements and themes in individual interviews as they were transcribed. While the study was initially proposed in my research practicum as a critical ethnography, I had not yet identified a specific phenomenological lens through which to interpret the findings. For the purposes of the practicum, it had been enough to identify the questions I wanted to address as best addressed by a qualitative design and to explore a particular type of design. Up until this point, I had not considered the lack of a specific phenomenological lens a problem. But to analyze my data, more specificity was necessary to achieve the rigor required for dissertation work. And that is when the summer of kissing frogs began, and you already know the happy ending! So how did my summer fling with Alfred Schutz lead to a deep and meaningful relationship that resulted in a fall and winter of data analysis, once my committee had fully approved the work I had done during my dissertation seminar over the summer?

While reviewing the transcripts of participant interviews, I was also wrestling at the same time with Schutz's concepts of social phenomenology, and I started to see how those concepts would bring clarity and meaning to the data. I had spent the summer writing a broad outline of Schutz's theory, concepts, and definitions that I felt were relevant to the aim of my study and the questions I had asked. Some of these concepts included *biographically determined situations, intersubjectivity, historicity, personal orientation, relevances, transcendence, symbols, typifications, we-relationships, group status,* and *equality* (Schutz, 1962, 1964). These concepts resonated with the theory underlying critical ethnographic design. I kept a journal as I developed my understanding of Schutz's work and of how concepts and definitions of social phenomenology related to health care, health care roles, and health care relationships. Every few days, I had my husband read my journal and provide feedback. He would often say something like, "I don't think you have a clear understanding of the distinction between signs and symbols. Maybe you should go back and reread some of what Schutz wrote about that"; or "there is not the same negative value associated with *typification* as there is with *stereotyping,* so try not to conceptualize typification as a negative thing … it is just a way of making sense of the world." It was like having a committee member in residence.

When I began data analysis in the fall, I chose to use Graneheim and Lundman's (2004) qualitative content analysis method to meet Lincoln and Guba's (1985) trustworthiness criteria. Graneheim and Lundman (2004) specifically used the trustworthiness criteria in the development of their analytic method. They adhered to the basic premise that qualitative data collection requires mutuality between researcher and participant, and that any content, whether interviews, observations, or records review, contains many meanings; they also relied heavily on application of communication theory to justify their approach.

Graneheim and Lundman (2004) offered several quite different examples of how their system can be applied. They argued that using their system will specifically address credibility, dependability, and transferability, thereby establishing trustworthiness as defined by Lincoln and Guba (1985). The beauty of the method is that it is quite flexible and can be used in many different ways. When I decided that it would be most relevant to analyze and interpret the data through a Schutzian lens, Graneheim and Lundman's (2004) method was quite useful to me in organizing and defining broader content areas, categories, and codes at the beginning of data analysis, and more as a processual reference and support as I wrestled with the more abstract themes.

I had really begun data analysis by listening to each recorded unit of analysis, or interview, within a week of its occurrence, and making casual notes in my research journal about topics or comments that seemed to reflect manifest and latent content directly related to the research questions. After each interview was completed and I had made initial notes, it was transcribed into a hard copy. These interviews occurred during the spring and summer of 2011 and were transcribed subsequently. Later that fall, as I read each hard copy, I highlighted what I felt were relevant meaning units and created a subset of interview documents that included only those words, sentences, or paragraphs containing meaning relevant to the content and context of the study's purpose and the overarching theoretical frameworks of race, ethnicity, culture, social justice, and critical theory. After reading through the interview subsets several times, I established two major content areas based on the subsets—(a) relevant precursors to health care encounters and (b) encounters with health care professionals— and assigned codes to these content areas that would be consistent with Alfred Schutz's social phenomenology. I then read through the data subsets again and, using condensation and abstraction, established codes for specific categorical threads that ran throughout the data in each of the two major content areas.

At this point, it was necessary to return to each fully transcribed interview to see if I had missed relevant data when I created the subsets. At that time I added several other meaning units to the growing group of Schutzian codes and categories I had established within the content areas. These data were then analyzed and thematically interpreted within the framework of Alfred Schutz's social phenomenology. That the meaning units were so easily categorized was evidence that social phenomenology established a solid and appropriate foundation for finding meaning in this particular inquiry. When they were not easily categorized, I knew there was a processual problem: There were several instances during the analysis process in which my attempt to overcategorize either obscured important meaning or assigned meaning that did not exist. Recognition of this led me to create broader categories and subcategories and to be satisfied with allowing the data to speak.

Analysis of the coded data consisted of interpreting Schutzian themes that emerged from the coding process in light of the overarching theoretical frameworks of race, ethnicity, culture, social justice, and critical theory through what Munhall (2007) called discovery through writing. Indeed, van Manen (1990, p. 111) stated that "creating a phenomenological text is the object of the research process"; that writing is, in fact, the method and enables the writer to objectify thought and experience into an understanding of the world. Madison (2005) discussed the relational nature of writing, which considers the obligation to and care for not only the participants of the study but also the obligation to and care for the readers. Thus, the social phenomenology of Alfred Schutz, with its focus on the intersubjectivity of the social world, provided an interpretive framework for considering the experiences of African American parents in their children's health care encounters. Critical ethnography, with the dual components of ethnographic and critical analysis, was a useful methodological tool for analyzing these experiences within the Schutzian framework. The intense writing and analytical work that ensued throughout those fall and winter months (I estimate I spent approximately 200 hours doing data analysis and writing after the summer work was completed, not including later revisions required by my committee) culminated in the completion of the dissertation in the spring of 2012. I have since disseminated some of the findings of my dissertation work in the form of podium presentations at several international nursing conferences and as recommendations in the first chapter of an edited volume about chronic illness (Stoltzfus, Green, & Schumm, 2013).

So what is the moral of this story? There are two lessons the princess learned in the various iterations of the tale of the princess and the frog, that the novice researcher may also learn in his or her quest for the right phenomenologist to frame a qualitative inquiry: (a) Superficial activity and facile commitments made at the side of the phenomenological pond did not result in an understanding of the frog's true nature. Only after some difficult dwelling with commitment, unpleasantness, difficulty, and engagement did the princess understand the frog's character. This was true of my own experience with phenomenology and, particularly, of Alfred Schutz. It is not possible to understand phenomenology only in a categorical sense, well enough to use as a foundation for a study. It is imperative to read broadly enough to see the differences among various phenomenological approaches and deeply enough to be able to find a phenomenologist whose work resonates with the aim of the particular study. This broad and deep understanding may only be gained through commitment, (some) unpleasantness, difficulty, and engagement. (b) There are parent figures in these tales, one a benevolent but authoritative father who reminds the princess to fulfill her promises, another an ailing mother who has sent her daughters in search of a cure from a well. In either case, it is the behest of a parent that propels an unwilling child to pursue a distasteful relationship. What could this paternalistic lesson possibly teach emancipated nursing researchers? In the scholarly disciplines, there exist evolving standards of rigor or quality that the researcher is expected to observe, though there may be some disagreement about what these standards are (Emden & Sandelowski, 1998; Sandelowski, 1993; Thorne, 2011; Thorne, Reimer Kirkham, & O'Flynn-Magee, 2004; Whittemore, Chase, & Mandle, 2001); and I would argue that these existing standards or paradigms are representative of the parent figures in the tale. And there is some question about how emancipated we, in the academy, actually are (Watkins, 2012; Yee, 2011), and so I will argue that the lesson holds sound and true. The Western research paradigm remains heavily influenced by positivism and, though admittedly changing, fairly rigid. This is evident in the expectations of writers and scholars when submitting proposals for dissertations and publications. Being a lover of structure and rules, this does not present a problem for me, but then, I come from a culture in which I also heard and read the tale of the princess and the frog many times as I was growing up, so the lessons made sense to me, and this lesson made particular sense: Meet the expectations and standards for rigor and quality set forth by your discipline and by the academy. I committed myself to those strategies recommended by my professors and by committee members, and in the scholarly literature. I adhered carefully to the processes and timelines required by my institution. While some of the activities seemed tedious (as in the maintenance of a research journal), in retrospect they most often proved invaluable, and established good habits. Yes, "good habits" are a matter of opinion; but if you are reading this book, my guess is that you have already adopted the narrative that has dictated what these are. But that is a rather cynical sentiment and the reader requires a happy ending.

And so, let me end with a short paragraph about Alfred Schutz, who was actually "not a frog, but a prince with beautiful friendly eyes. And he was now, according to her father's will, her dear companion" (Grimm & Grimm, 1812). Alfred Schutz's work, social phenomenology, uniquely situated in human relationships and in how people typify situations, experiences, and one another based on their biographically determined situations, is quite relevant for nursing's concerns with the concepts of person, nursing, health, and environment and the interactions among them:

But the order of Nature and of Society is common to all mankind [*sic*]. It furnishes to everyone the setting of the cycle of his individual life, of birth, aging, death, health and sickness, hopes and fears. Each of us participates in the recurrent rhythm of nature; to each of us the movements of the sun and moon and stars, the change between day and night, and the cycle of the seasons are elements of his [*sic*] situation. (Schutz, 1962, p. 330)

Alfred Schutz's social phenomenology is particularly appropriate for nursing, and is perhaps underutilized. I believe great opportunities exist for broadening the scope and application of social phenomenology in nursing research.

REFERENCES

Barber, M. (2011). Alfred Schutz. In E. N. Zalta (Ed.), *The Stanford encyclopedia of philosophy*. Retrieved from the Stanford University website http://plato.stanford.edu/archives/sum2011/entries/schutz/
Beneloiel, J. (1984). Advancing nursing science: Qualitative approaches. *Western Journal of Nursing Research in Nursing and Health, 7,* 1–8.
Bryman, A. (2004). *Social research methods*. Oxford, UK: Oxford University Press.
Campbell, J. F. (1969). The tale of the queen who sought a drink from a certain well. *Popular tales of the West Highlands: Orally collected*. Detroit, MI: Singing Tree Press.
Creswell, J. (2007). *Qualitative inquiry and research design: Choosing among five approaches*. Thousand Oaks, CA: Sage Publications.
Czarniawska, B. (2004). *Narratives in social science research*. London, UK: Sage.
Dombro, M. (2007). Historical and philosophical foundations of qualitative research. In P. Munhall (Ed.), *Nursing research: A qualitative perspective*. Sudbury, MA: Jones and Bartlett.
Duffy, M. (2007). Narrative inquiry: The method. In P. Munhall (Ed.), *Nursing research: A qualitative perspective* (pp. 421–440). Sudbury, MA: Jones and Bartlett.
Emden, C., & Sandelowski, M. (1998). The good, the bad and the relative, part one: Conceptions of goodness in qualitative research. *International Journal of Nursing Practice, 4,* 206–212. doi:10.1046/j.1440-172X.1998.00105.x
Graneheim, U., & Lundman, B. (2004). Qualitative concept analysis in nursing research: Concepts, procedures and measures to achieve trustworthiness. *Nurse Education Today, 24,* 105–112.
Green, R. (2012). *African American parents' experiences in their children's health care encounters* (Dissertations, Theses and Capstone Projects). Paper 498. Retrieved from http://digitalcommons.kennesaw.edu/cgi/viewcontent.cgi?article=1498&context=etd

Grimm. J., & Grimm, W. (1812). The frog king. (D. L. Ashliman, Trans.). Retrieved from www.pitt.edu/~dash/grimm001.html

Guest, G., Namey, E., & Mitchell, M. (2013). *Collecting qualitative data: A field manual for applied research*. Thousand Oaks, CA: Sage.

International Association for the Study of the Philosophy of Edith Stein (IASPES). (2009). Academic biography. Retrieved from www.edithsteincircle.com

Janesick, V. (1994). The dance of qualitative research design: Metaphor, methodolatry and meaning. In N. K. Denzin & Y. S. Lincoln (Eds.), *Handbook of qualitative research* (pp. 209–219). Thousand Oaks, CA: Sage.

Kincheloe, J., & Berry, K. (2004). *Rigour and complexity in educational research: Conceptualizing the bricolage*. Berkshire, UK: Open University Press.

Lincoln, Y., & Guba, E. (1985). *Naturalistic inquiry*. Beverly Hills, CA: Sage.

Madison, D. (2005). *Critical ethnography: Method, ethics, and performance*. Thousand Oaks, CA: Sage.

Martin, G. (2013). *The meaning and origin of the expression: A woman needs a man like a fish needs a bicycle*. Retrieved from The Phrasefinder website at http://www.phrases.org.uk/meanings/414150.html

Munhall, P. (2007). *Nursing research: A qualitative perspective*. Sudbury, MA; Jones and Bartlett.

National Institutes of Health. (2008). Guidelines for scientific record keeping in the Intramural Research Program at the NIH. Retrieved from http://sourcebook.od.nih.gov/ethic-conduct/recordkeeping.pdf

Ortlipp, M. (2008). Keeping and using reflective journals in the qualitative research process. *The Qualitative Report, 13*(4), 695–705.

Sandelowski, M. (1993). Rigor or rigor mortis: The problem of rigor in qualitative research revisited. *Advances in Nursing Science, 16*, 1–8.

Schutz, A. (1962). *The problem of social reality: Collected papers one*. The Hague, The Netherlands: Martinus Nijhoff.

Schutz, A. (1964). *Collected papers two: Studies in social theory*. The Hague, The Netherlands: Martinus Nijhoff.

Stein, E., & Stein, W. (1989). *On the problem of empathy: The collected works of Edith Stein*. Washington, DC: ICS Publications.

Stoltzfus, M. (1998). *Moral manifestation: Alfred Schutz's contributions to the study of moral agency in the social world*. Nashville, TN: Vanderbilt University.

Stoltzfus, M., Green, R., & Schumm, D. (2013). *Chronic illness, spirituality, and healing: Diverse disciplinary, religious, and cultural perspectives*. New York, NY: Palgrave Macmillan.

Thomas, J. (1993). *Doing critical ethnography*. Newbury Park, CA: Sage.

Thorne, S. (2011). Toward methodological emancipation in applied health research. *Qualitative Health Research, 21*(4), 443–453. doi:10.1177/1049732310392595

Thorne, S., Reimer Kirkham, S., & O'Flynn-Magee, K. (2004). The analytic challenge in interpretive description. *International Journal of Qualitative Methods, 3*(1). Article 1. Retrieved from https://ejournals.library.ualberta.ca/index.php/IJQM/article/view/4481/3619

Tillman, L. (2002). Culturally sensitive research approaches: An African American perspective. *Educational Researcher, 31*(9), 3–12.

van Manen, M. (1990). *Researching lived experience.* Ontario, Canada: Althouse Press.

Watkins, B. (2012). It's time for Black scholars to escape the academic plantation [blog]. Retrieved from http://www.yourblackworld.net/2012/04/featured-bloggers/dr-boyce-its-time-for-black-scholars-to-escape-the-academic-plantation/

Whittemore, R., Chase, S., & Mandle, C. (2001). Pearls, pith, and provocation: Validity in qualitative research. *Qualitative Health Research, 11*(4), 522–537.

Yee, J. (2011). *Feminism for real: Deconstructing the academic industrial complex of feminism.* Ottawa, Ontario, Canada: Canadian Centre for Policy Alternatives.

THE VALUE OF DIALOGUE WHEN PLANNING AND CONDUCTING PHENOMENOLOGICAL RESEARCH: REFLECTIONS OF A DISSERTATION CHAIR AND DOCTORAL STUDENT

Joan Such Lockhart and Lenore K. Resick

Whether you are a novice or an experienced researcher, engaging in an open dialogue with other scholars when developing and conducting a study enables you to gain multiple perspectives regarding the proposed topic and research method. The importance of using dialogue as a teaching–learning strategy is most apparent when mentoring new researchers who are beginning their research trajectories. This chapter provides the personal reflections (exchanges) between a dissertation chair and a doctoral student who conducted a hermeneutic phenomenological study about the meaning of health among midlife Russian-speaking women.

In this chapter, we attempt to retrace the dialogue that occurred at select key points during the dissertation process: (a) choosing a dissertation topic and committee, (b) preparing the research proposal, (c) collecting and analyzing data, and (d) disseminating study results. We hope this chapter helps other researchers as they mentor future researchers. In fact, we plan to use this chapter ourselves to help our students better understand the dissertation "journey" and the decisions, issues, and challenges they may encounter, along with creative solutions. *Note:* In this chapter, Dr. Lenore K. Resick (LKR) provides the doctoral student's perspective, while Dr. Joan Such Lockhart (JSL) offers reflections in the dissertation chair role.

DESCRIPTION OF THE STUDY

This study, "The Meaning of Health among Midlife Russian-Speaking Women," was completed and published in the *Journal of Nursing Scholarship* (Resick, 2008). Readers are referred to this source for a full description of the study, which was the second author's dissertation. The purpose was to explore the phenomenon of health among midlife Russian-speaking women from the former Soviet Union (FSU) by interviewing 12 women aged 40 to 61 who spoke English and immigrated to the United States after 1991. A hermeneutical approach was used to analyze the data. The interviews generated the following themes: health as being highly valued, though less of a priority during immigration; being a stranger and seeking the familiar; grieving a loss and building a new life; experiencing changes and transitions; trusting self; and the importance of hope.

It was concluded that, although health was less of a priority during the immigration process, the women valued and were knowledgeable about health, participated in self-care practices, trusted their own abilities to make self-care decisions, and sought health-related information. This is a vulnerable population at risk for the onset of chronic medical conditions associated with the process of aging, past exposures, the tendency to avoid health screening, and current stressors related to immigration and family responsibilities. Implications include the need for interventions to build trust, to assess self-care practices, and to understand values and beliefs concerning health screening. Future research recommendations include replication with other samples within this population and exploring curative beliefs and practices more fully. Ultimately, this study design could be applied to other immigrant populations in Western cultures. Midlife Russian-speaking women from the FSU are a vulnerable group at risk for the onset of chronic medical conditions associated with aging, past exposures, the tendency to avoid health screening, and current stressors related to immigration and family responsibilities (Resick, 2008).

CHOOSING A DISSERTATION TOPIC AND CHAIR

LKR: I chose to focus on health and Russian-speaking women through my clinical encounters with this population. For several months I volunteered as a nurse practitioner in an outreach program offering health information and free screening mammograms to new Americans living in my home community. The majority of this population was middle-aged Russian-speaking women who recently migrated from Eastern Europe with refugee status. Very few women took advantage of these services. I began talking to the women. Some spoke fluent English and some required the assistance of an interpreter. I asked about perceptions of wellness and health. My interpreter was quick to point out to me that there was no one word for "wellness" that translated from English to Russian. She went on to say, "it is very complicated . . . it will be hard for you to understand this unless you are a Russian." During this same time period, unrelated to my volunteer work, I had the opportunity to travel to Russia as a visiting professor twice over a 2-year period. I kept a journal during my travels in Russia. In this journal, I found myself writing this same phrase after asking my nurse colleagues and Russian hosts about health and health care in Russia. The common response was "it is very complicated . . . it will be hard for you to understand unless you are a Russian." Through my unique experience to carry out preliminary field work in the culture of origin as well as the culture of destination, I grew to value the importance of understanding the meaning of interpretation of a phenomenon within the context of culture and lived history of the individual. I returned to the United States knowing that I had to find out more about the meaning of health for the Russian-speaking women who had migrated to my community.

Although I already had a dissertation topic that focused on health of midlife women, after my return from Russia, I knew that the focus on the Russian-speaking women would be of great value to understanding why the current screening health services that were available and accessible to the population were underused. For me to follow through with the research question that centered on understanding the women, I sought out a chair for my committee who had an understanding of cross-cultural health issues and qualitative methods. Although I knew that a qualitative design would best serve my interest, I did not have my question in a final format, so I was not sure which method would best fit. I sought the advice of Dr. Joan Such Lockhart, who had experience in qualitative designs, specifically hermeneutic phenomenology. While reading through the literature, I learned of Dr. Julienne Lipson's ethnographic studies of Russian-speaking populations. I sought the expertise of both researchers, who generously gave their time to discuss my topic of interest and mentor me through the dissertation process.

JSL: Over the past 15 years of teaching in our PhD nursing program, it has been my experience that, although all applicants propose a general "topic area" for their dissertation research, very few applicants have yet had the opportunity (or ability) to systematically search the research literature to identify potential gaps that need to be addressed. As with Dr. Resick, whose international experience sparked the beginning of her interest in the health needs of midlife women, topics proposed by other applicants often emerge from their clinical practice, teaching, and/or personal interests.

It has been evident over recent years that increasing numbers of applicants have "done their homework" when preparing their application to the PhD program by searching our school's website and identifying faculty with similar research interests or expertise. Dr. Resick described the process that she used to select her dissertation chair and members. I had been fortunate to have been mentored by Dr. Marlene Zichi Cohen, a nationally known expert in hermeneutic phenomenology, during a previous study in head and neck oncology. Similar to Dr. Resick's account, I located Dr. Cohen through a literature search. Since our doctoral program has been offered online since 1997, students have had the advantage of inviting researchers around the world to serve as external members on their dissertation committees.

PREPARING THE RESEARCH PROPOSAL

Reviewing the Literature and Conceptual Issues

LKR: I reviewed the literature a priori and after the data were generated. The literature review included a historical and current view of the experiences of Eastern European immigrants/refugees to Western cultures and the health experiences of immigrants/refugees who came from Russian-speaking cultures and settled in Western countries. I included studies in English from Israel, Australia, and other Western cultures. I also reviewed studies involving immigrants and refugees from other cultures who settled in Western countries. I learned that each wave of refugees and immigrants have a history and a culture within a culture that was often not addressed in the studies I reviewed. After the data for my study were generated, I went back to the literature and searched for studies related to health and the meaning of health from other waves of immigrants and refugees from Russian-speaking cultures.

JSL: Some phenomenological sources suggest that researchers should review the literature in depth only *after* data are collected. However, it is important for students to become familiar with the research, not only to clarify the problem and its significance for future study, but also to realize the research gaps in the topic in developing a proposal. Dr. Resick describes the thorough literature review that she conducted prior to conducting the study. Her review helped her identify what was already known about the proposed topic, what was unknown, and what gaps needed to be addressed. After completing the data analysis, Dr. Resick return to her prior literature review and searched the research as new themes were generated.

Justifying Significance

LKR: I was working with the population who did not use the health screenings offered to them to the extent that was expected by the local health care facilities. By speaking with the women in my role as a nurse practitioner, I learned that the women were the gatekeepers for family members in need of health care. I also heard from the Russian-speaking women in the United States the same phrase my interpreter used for health in Russia: "it is complicated . . . ." Understanding the meaning of health for midlife Russian-speaking women was important to the women not only when deciding to seek screening and health care but also to the health of their family. In my search of the literature, I found conflicting reports regarding the utilization of health care services by new immigrants and refugees. I could not find one study that addressed the health beliefs of midlife Russian-speaking women. The local, state, and regional census data did not include this population. I could find no statistics on the number of refugees/immigrants from Eastern Europe in the area where I was interested in conducting the research. In addition, the literature was lacking the voices of this population expressing their own perspectives about the meaning of health in the context of immigration. As a result, this group was relatively silent and invisible. The census data showed that, unlike other waves of émigrés to the United States, a large number of this wave of émigrés were midlife women. My rationale for choosing this age group was based on my experience as a nurse practitioner. I knew that midlife for women is not only associated with menopause but also the onset of chronic diseases that are modifiable if diagnosed early enough and often preventable. To learn about their meaning of health would help me understand the best approaches to implement effective prevention and disease management interventions. The literature argues that effective interventions must be acceptable, accessible, and culturally appropriate to the population (Meleis et al., 1995). I justified the significance by my experience as a health care provider in giving voice to a voiceless group in the community.

JSL: When doctoral students are preparing their topic for approval and/or their research proposal, it is essential for them to identify the problem and its significance—the "so what?" for proposing their research study. Dr. Resick addressed the significance of her proposed study through her observations in clinical practice and her review of relevant research on the topic.

Choosing the Methodology

LKR: I used a hermeneutic/phenomenological approach in my study since I wanted to understand health from the perspective of the women in the context of the wave of immigration they were experiencing. In addition, I was aware of the challenges of maintaining a culturally competent approach throughout the research process. Although culture and social issues are part of the experiences, they were not the focus of the question. By this I mean that I tried to remain focused on the lived experience of health as described by the women in the context of the immigration experience. From the literature, I learned that an essential aspect of the hermeneutic approach is looking "with" the other at what is being communicated rather than looking "at" the person who is communicating (Gadamer, 1977). I sought to understand and validate the responses of the study participants and to seek confirmation and clarification of their interpretations throughout the research process. My research question involved seeking to understand the meaning of health from the perspectives of the Russian-speaking women. A hermeneutic approach in the research design provides understanding; in contrast, empirical methods provide explanations. Of interest, many of the women I interviewed were familiar with quantitative methods in their homeland and found my qualitative approach a novelty. One participant asked if she could come to my dissertation defense. She sat in the back of the room and, after the defense was over, validated everything I presented.

My research approach followed the Dutch phenomenology of the "Utrecht School" (Barritt, Beekman, Bleeker, & Mulderij, 1983, 1984, 1985). This approach best met both aspects of descriptive and interpretive phenomenology (Cohen & Omery, 1994; van Manen, 2014). I felt that I needed to guide the research process, which would focus on what participants expressed regarding the meaning of health within the context of immigration. Before I started any of the interviews, I wrote down the presuppositions that I would be discussing with the participants in my journal. I analyzed my responses to be sure my preconceptions to the answers did not influence the responses I received from the participants during the study (Cohen, 1995).

I chose this design over other qualitative designs because of my experience in Russia and the phrase that I kept hearing, "it is complicated . . . it will be hard for you to understand this unless you are a Russian." It became very clear to me that translation and interpretation were contextual and, at times, there was no one word of equal translation. One example was the English word "wellness": The translation to Russian required my interpreter to use several sentences in Russian to put the meaning into a Russian context. By using the Dutch approach that supported features of descriptive and interpretive phenomenology expressed within a context, I was better able to capture the responses of the participants within a context and the meaning of these expressions and actions within the context of migration. The interpretive process in this study allowed time for me to dialogue with the participants and discuss interpretations, verify meanings, and document the outcomes of our discussion (Resick, 2006).

JSL: Anecdotally, some students have voiced their preference for a specific research design—quantitative, qualitative, or a mixture—shortly after they have completed one or more of their methods courses. Unfortunately, their premature decisions are often made without having completed a thorough review of the research on their topic and/or identifying a clear research purpose/questions/aims. In some cases, students' rationale for choosing a "qualitative" method may not be supported (e.g., they think the process is faster using a qualitative vs. a quantitative method, they feel uncomfortable using statistics, etc.). In this case, Dr. Resick was strongly supported in her decision not only to use a qualitative approach to answer her research question but also to defend her choice of hermeneutic phenomenology over other qualitative methods (ethnography, grounded theory, etc.).

Selecting and Recruiting Participants

LKR: The participants were recruited by purposive sampling and snowballing. I was actively involved as a nurse practitioner in the Russian community for about 5 years prior to conducting the study. I talked to two Russian-speaking women who recognized me from my volunteer work and who were well respected by the Russian community. These women understood the purpose of the study and supported the need for the study for better communication among health care providers and new arrivals to the Russian community in the area. As I interviewed more women, I asked them to identify and refer women who met the inclusion criteria to me. I also put flyers in English and Russian on library bulletin boards, supermarket community boards, community organizations, health care provider waiting rooms, city newspapers, synagogues, church bulletins, hospitals, and local universities. I wanted to be sure the recruitment flyers were in a variety of settings in order to attract a variety of study participants with maximum variation (Resick, 2006).

I had originally set the age range for participants to be 40 to 60 years of age as inclusion criteria for the study. Since one of the women who was

61 years of age met all other criteria for the study, I included her interviews in the study, as the analysis of these transcripts did not change the findings from the other interviews. Originally, my inclusion criteria included women who had been in the United States for less than 10 years. I used 10 years because the literature identified this as the time period when immigrants became acculturated to the culture of the destination (Leclere, Jensen, & Biddlecom, 1994). During the interview process, I learned from the study participants that it was more important to consider migration of this group as those women migrating to the United States after the fall of the FSU (in 1991) as the inclusion criteria and not the 10-year period as noted in the literature.

I continued my interviews until no new themes were identified through data analysis. My study included 12 women who were interviewed twice. The study took place over a period of 6 months.

JSL: Gaining access to a sufficient pool of subjects (participants) who meet the inclusion criteria for a qualitative study is often a challenge in any research, regardless of the study method. However, recruiting participants for a phenomenological study in which the researcher is asking them to not only share personal accounts of their "lived experience," but to also audio-tape the interview, requires a great deal of advance thought and planning on the part of the researcher.

Dr. Resick explained how she gained entry into the community of Russian immigrant women over time in her role as a clinician. She had created a sense of trust with the informal gatekeepers within the community who referred her to other potential participants. Also, the gatekeepers supported the need for the study and its importance for the health of the current and future women in the community. It was apparent that Dr. Resick had access to sufficient numbers of participants to reach saturation (Cohen, Kahn, & Steeves, 2000). In my experience, students often realize the true meaning of "saturation" only after they actually experience it in the field.

Obtaining Institutional Review Board Approval

LKR: In this study I used pseudonyms. I learned from one of the gatekeepers to the Russian-speaking community that it would not be unusual for the participants to decline being audiotaped. In preparation for refusal to be taped, I offered both the audiotape and note taking to the participants. No one declined being audiotaped. I removed all identifying information from the transcripts and assigned pseudonyms. I asked a gatekeeper to the community to give me example of Russian names for women. I started to de-identify the first interview with a Russian name that began with "A," then the next interview I de-identified with a name that began with "B," and continued until "L" in order to give all 12 participants a de-identified Russian name. I would not use pseudonyms in future studies. I did not think about this, but in another study of Iraqi refugees that I co-authored and submitted for review a few years after publishing my dissertation, the reviewers requested that I not use pseudonyms because of the possibility of putting the participants at risk for false identification. I tend to de-identify using numbers now.

The audiotapes, journal, and all materials related to the study were kept in a locked drawer in my home office. I also kept a journal in my purse and by my bed since I found that I kept thinking of the study throughout the day and would wake up thinking of ideas that I needed to write down so as not to forget them.

JSL: Preserving the anonymity of participants is essential in conducting phenomenological research, especially when they are sharing their personal perspectives. As Dr. Resick mentions, careful attention to the data management according to institutional review board (IRB) guidelines is vital. It is evident in this account that the researcher often "lives" the study as well.

COLLECTING AND ANALYZING DATA

Choosing the Appropriate Setting for Data Collection

LKR: Since all the women I interviewed were working outside the home, I made an effort to arrange the interviews around the work schedules of the women and in a private place of their choice. Most of the interviews took place during the day and occurred over tea and sometimes over a meal in the participant's home. Before I left for an interview, I called my dissertation chair so she would know where I was going, and I called her once the interview was done. The location for the study was based on the large influx of Russian-speaking immigrants to the region, and the state was one of the top 10 states in the United States with the largest foreign-born population from Russian-speaking countries. I could find no literature about the group that settled in this region.

JSL: Privacy is a priority when conducting audiotaped interviews in phenomenological research, so the researcher needs to carefully choose a location that is agreeable to both the participant and the researcher. Although we paid attention to ensuring a "private" interview, we later realized that we needed to consider potential safety issues, not only for the participants but also for Dr. Resick, who was alone in participants' homes whose locations were unknown to anyone. It was also important for Dr. Resick to decide, in advance, if she would limit the interview session to only the participant and herself or if others would be allowed to be present. She needed to anticipate the impact of having the additional person present during the interview on the study findings.

Challenges Encountered During the Interview Process

LKR: Before starting the interview, I asked permission to tape the interview. I asked the question again when I turned the tape on so that I had a record of the permission. I reviewed my role as a nurse researcher and how it was different from my role as a clinical practitioner. One of the challenges I faced was how to separate my role as clinician from my role as researcher. I found that this worked best for me by discussing with the participants at the start of the interview that once the interview was over, I would answer health-related questions that were part of my role as clinician.

I created a demographic questionnaire as a guide to collect information about age, length of time in the United States, location of homeland, marital status, number of children, type of work they did in the homeland, and type of work they do now in the United States. I piloted this tool on a gatekeeper from the community before using it in the study. Since the goal of the interview was to ask the questions that would lead to the meaning of health within the context of the immigration experience, I used an open-ended interview guide that included the question "Tell me what health means to you."

I learned very quickly that data collection using the personal and informal approach brought about a discussion of issues of importance to the participants and led the discussion to topics of interest to the study participants. This discussion resulted in rich data that were not the focus of the research questions. This was also the experience of the third member of my committee, who conducted a study of Bosnian and Russian-speaking refugees who settled in the West Coast (Lipson, Weinstein, Gladstone, & Sarnoff, 2003).

My study was of interest to a local agency that provided funding for projects aimed at the Russian-speaking immigrant community. I was approached by this local funding organization who served this population about submitting a proposal for the funding for my study. To receive funding from this agency, the requirement was that I ask specific interview questions the potential funders requested about study participants. Since the research requirements for the funding were not congruent with the research question, method, and design I had chosen, I declined to submit a funding proposal, and thus retained the trust of many in this immigrant population. I was glad I made the decision not to change my research question or method to meet the funding requirements, since I realized from study participants that being associated with this agency could have resulted in lack of trust in me as the researcher and skewed or missing data in the interviews.

Even though I had a plan regarding how to separate my clinician role from the researcher role, I found it a challenge at times to hold back my clinician self and maintain the researcher role during the interview process. As the women expressed their experiences and meaning of health, I found myself wanting to jump into health teaching or move the interview toward asking more direct diagnostic questions instead of letting the women guide the interviews and listening to the voices of the émigrés. My dissertation chair listened to my first set of interviews and pointed out areas in which I could improve my interview technique and maintain the role of researcher. She spot-checked the interviews after that time to ensure the fidelity of the interviewing process.

Data were collected within a 6-month period. The timeline for analysis required more time than I had anticipated. In my master's program, I learned to analyze data manually using colored highlighters. For this piece of research, along with the manual method, I used a software package to organize my data. Learning the software was extremely time consuming and expensive.

JSL: When choosing the interview question(s) for a hermeneutic phenomenological study, there are several things that students often misunderstand. First, it is important that the student realizes that the research question is different from the data collection tool or the interview questions. Second, the interview questions need to be open-ended and semistructured. It is important that the participant and the participant's responses, and not the researcher, guide the interview. The researcher's role involves active listening and the use of probes to encourage the participant to elaborate on the response and, perhaps, provide an example or situation that best illustrates the participant's perspective. The researcher needs to practice the interview process and the use of the audiotape recorder. Field notes should be recorded either during the interview (sometimes difficult) or immediately after the interview. Dr. Resick provided an example of this.

Since data analysis and data collection are conducted concurrently, it is helpful for students to develop an appropriate timeline to accommodate these research phases. Students often underestimate the amount of time that needs to be dedicated to the interviews and especially time needed for data analysis. Similar to Dr. Resick, students use software products to manage the interview data. However, it is important for students to plan in advance for time and the location to receive such training and practice.

Dr. Resick mentioned a challenge that she encountered while she was conducting the interviews—differentiating and acting from the clinician's role versus the researcher's role. It is important to anticipate this situation in advance with students and discuss appropriate behaviors.

Data Analysis

LKR: Data were member-checked with study participants at a second interview to validate responses and identify themes. In my journal I kept notes about my experience as the researcher and how I was influenced by the study participants. Intercoder reliability was achieved by another qualitative researcher coding transcripts and coming together to discuss if we had come to similar or identical thematic analysis of the transcripts. Recorded interviews were critiqued by my chair to check for leading questioning. Data were also collected within a 6-month period to decrease the chance of the interview process changing over an extended period of time (Tripp-Reimer, 1985).

JSL: Ensuring the quality of phenomenological research is essential. Students need to identify specific strategies that they will follow during the research process to ensure the study's trustworthiness or rigor (Lincoln & Guba, 1985). As Dr. Resick explained, she developed mechanisms for maintaining the study's credibility, transferability, dependability, and confirmability (Lincoln & Guba, 1985).

DISSEMINATING THE STUDY FINDINGS

LKR: Acceptance for publication was nearly a 6-month process. The manuscript was published after a round of review of two different reviewers and suggested changes. Qualitative studies of this population in Western countries were very scarce. The manuscript was valuable because Russian-speaking women left their homeland for other Western cultures after the fall of the FSU, and little was written about this phenomenon to prepare health care providers in other Western nations for this influx of new émigrés from the FSU. This study provided a description and interpretation of health for these women within the context of the vulnerable time of resettlement. It was a challenge to get 283 pages of the dissertation down to a 21-page manuscript. The feedback I received from the reviewers was invaluable to me. Their feedback helped me realize that what was clear to me may not be clear to others. For example, one reviewer felt I needed more information about the participants. Another felt there should be more emphasis on the findings and that I had condense the method and design to be able to do this within the page limits.

JSL: Preparing for the final dissertation defense presents a challenge for doctoral students, especially when reporting on a phenomenological study with large amounts of information in the Findings and Discussion portions of the dissertation. Therefore, students often need help in preparing the presentation within a limited time. This same challenge occurs with publishing the study in peer-reviewed journals. In this latter case, it is often helpful to advise students to seek sample articles that reported on phenomenological studies in the journal of their choice to follow as a template. Dr. Resick was very successful in her publishing efforts, despite the two rounds of reviewers' comments. She chose a high-quality journal and emphasized the significance of her work to the advancement of nursing knowledge.

SUMMARY

In closing, planning and conducting a hermeneutic phenomenological study and engaging in an open dialogue between/among researchers is a valuable practice that supports the significance of the findings. In the situation presented in this chapter, ongoing communication between the dissertation chair and student in order to anticipate and manage possible challenges and issues was essential to the decision-making process and study findings.

REFERENCES

Barritt, L., Beekman, T., Bleeker, H., & Mulderij, K. J. (1983). *A handbook for phenomenological research in education.* Ann Arbor, MI: University of Michigan.

Barritt, L., Beekman, T., Bleeker, H., & Mulderij, K. J. (1984). Analyzing phenomenological descriptions. *Phenomenology + Pedagogy, 2*(1), 1–17.

Barritt, L., Beekman, T., Bleeker, H., & Mulderij, K. J. (1985). *Researching education practice.* Grand Forks, ND: Center for Teaching & Learning, University of North Dakota.

Cohen, M. Z. (1995). The experience of surgery: Phenomenological clinical nursing research. In A. Omery, C. Kasper, & G. Page (Eds.), *In search of nursing science* (pp. 159–174). Thousand Oaks, CA: Sage.

Cohen, M. Z., Kahn, D. I., & Steeves, R. H. (2000). *Hermeneutic phenomenological research: A practical guide for nurse researchers.* Thousand Oaks, CA: Sage.

Cohen, M. Z., & Omery, A. (1994). Schools of phenomenology: Implications for research. In J. M. Morse (Ed.), *Critical issues in qualitative research* (pp. 136–156). Thousand Oaks, CA: Sage.

Gadamer, H. (1977). Editor's introduction. In Linge, D. E. (Trans. & Ed.), *Philosophical hermeneutics* (pp. vii–viii). Berkeley, CA: University of California Press.

LeClere, F., Jensen, L., & Biddlecom, A. E. (1994). Health care utilization, family context, and adaptation among immigrants to the United States. *Journal of Health and Social Behavior, 35*(4), 370–384.

Lincoln, Y., & Guba, E. (1985). *Naturalistic inquiry.* Thousand Oaks, CA: Sage.

Lipson, J. G., Weinstein, H. M., Gladstone, E. A., & Sarnoff, R. H. (2003). Bosnian and Soviet refugees' experience with health care. *Western Journal of Nursing Research, 25*(7), 854–871.

Meleis, A. I., Isenberg, M., Koerner, J. E., Lacey, B., & Stern, P. (1995). *Diversity marginalization, and culturally competent health care issues in knowledge development.* Washington, DC: American Academy of Nursing.

Resick, L. K. (2006). *The meaning of health among midlife Russian-speaking women* (Electronic dissertation). Duquesne University, Pittsburgh, PA.

Resick, L. K. (2008). The meaning of health among midlife Russian-speaking women. *Journal of Nursing Scholarship, 40*(3), 248–253.

Tripp-Reimer, T. (1985). Research in cultural diversity: Reliability issues in cross-cultural research. *Western Journal of Nursing Research, 7*(3), 391–392.

van Manen, M. (2014). *Phenomenology of practice: Meaning-giving methods in phenomenological research and writing (Developing qualitative inquiry).* Walnut Creek, CA: Left Coast Press.

CHAPTER SEVEN

USING PHENOMENOLOGY AS A RESEARCH METHOD IN COMMUNITY-BASED RESEARCH

Bonnie H. Bowie and Danuta Wojnar

DESCRIPTIVE PHENOMENOLOGY

Descriptive phenomenology research can be a very useful approach to learn about, better understand, and describe phenomena important to the human experience. In this chapter, lessons learned from the field are shared and guidelines are offered to assist prospective investigators considering phenomenology to guide community-based research.

Phenomenology is often considered central to the interpretive paradigm (LeVasseur, 2003; Lopez & Willis, 2004). For more than one hundred years, phenomenology has developed as a philosophical perspective and an approach to research (Tymieniecka, 2003). At the heart of phenomenology lies the researchers' attempt to describe and understand phenomena as experienced by individuals who have lived through them (Swanson & Wojnar, 2004). The two approaches that guide the majority of phenomenological investigations in nursing are descriptive and hermeneutic (interpretive) phenomenology. Both approaches are concerned with understanding the human experience; hence, they are considered by many to be foundational to nursing science. The philosophical basis and assumptions of descriptive phenomenology, which guided our research that explored Somali couples' parenting in the United States, are described in the subsequent paragraphs.

Edmund Husserl (1859–1938), a German philosopher and mathematician, is considered the founder of phenomenology as a philosophy and a descriptive (eidetic) approach to inquiry (Wojnar & Swanson, 2007). Husserl's central insight was that consciousness is the condition of all human experience. He wanted to explain how to overcome personal biases, which stand in the way of achieving the state of pure consciousness. These insights launched a new philosophy and a new approach to research (Moran, 2000).

In *Logical Investigations*, Husserl (1970) focused on exploring the concepts of human consciousness, intentionality, and the meaning of lived experience from the first-person perspective. The Husserlian approach to science assumed that the meaning of lived experiences may be best unraveled through one-to-one interactions between the researcher and the research participants, as well as through attentive listening and observation, to create representation of reality more refined than previous understandings (Husserl, 1970).

In subsequent works, Husserl (2001) presented a concept of transcendental subjectivity: a condition wherein the researcher can successfully abandon his or her own preconceived ideas and understandings and describe the phenomenon in its pure, universal sense. The state of transcendental subjectivity may be accomplished by employing the process called *bracketing*, also known as active stripping away of prior knowledge and personal bias so as not to influence the description of the phenomenon studied (Wojnar & Swanson, 2007). Bracketing has been described as (a) separating the phenomenon from the researcher's world and inspecting it; (b) dissecting the phenomenon to define it and analyze it; and (c) suspending all preconceptions regarding the phenomenon and seeking understanding through active listening, interaction with study participants, and analysis of the participants' stories (Giorgi, 2000). Some authors even proposed that researchers should withhold an in-depth literature review prior to conducting research in an attempt to neutralize bias and prior knowledge (Deutscher, 2001). Others have cautioned, however, that dismissing the literature limits the quality of research; in fact, some authors suggest that the literature itself may even serve as a source neutralizing personal bias (Swanson-Kauffman, 1986).

Husserl posits that, through bracketing, it is possible to gain insight into the common features of any lived experience. He referred to these features as universal essences or eidetic structures and considered them to represent the true nature of the phenomenon under investigation (Wojnar & Swanson, 2007). Hence, Husserl argued, if the description of lived experiences were to be considered generalizable, strict adherence to the principles of descriptive phenomenology must be employed to identify commonalities among research participants. Husserl also believed that human beings are agents responsible for influencing their environment. The converse, however, that the environment influences the lives and individual freedoms of people, was a peripheral concept to Husserl's beliefs (Deutscher, 2001).

In summary, descriptive phenomenology is a complex philosophical tradition and a research method. It requires investigation of phenomena through direct interactions with research participants. It calls upon investigators to set aside preconceptions through the procedures involved in bracketing (Wojnar & Swanson, 2007). As the researcher aims to define the phenomenon under investigation, he or she uses several frames of reference, including transcendental subjectivity (openness to the lived reality of others), eidetic essences (universalities), and interaction with study participants. The lived experience, as described by participants, is used to generate the universal structure of the phenomenon under study (Tymieniecka, 2003). The ultimate test of credibility of the descriptive phenomenological investigation's findings is the testimony from the participants themselves that the investigator's universal description of the phenomenon captured their personal experiences.

The steps of analysis considered essential in the descriptive phenomenological inquiry include (a) bracketing, (b) analyzing, (c) intuiting, and (d) describing (Colaizzi, 1978; Swanson-Kauffman & Schonwald, 1988). Although these steps are considered separate components of the descriptive phenomenological research method, each moment of the investigation is a blend of bracketing, analyzing, intuiting, and describing (Wojnar & Swanson, 2007). According to Wall, Glenn, Mitchinson, and Poole (2004), bracketing is an investigator's attempt to achieve a state of neutrality by putting aside biases and preconceptions about the phenomenon under investigation. Bracketing may be accomplished by a conscious attempt to neutralize it by keeping a self-reflective diary and field notes and seeking critique from methodological experts and individuals who are not research subjects but have professional expertise or personal knowledge of the phenomenon studied and by maintaining an ongoing notion about the role of personal bias throughout the data analysis process.

Rigorous analysis of data (analyzing) constitutes the second component of the descriptive phenomenological investigation. Colaizzi's (1978) method is commonly used to guide the analysis. It consists of the following seven steps (Colaizzi, 1978, pp. 48–71):

1. Reading and re-reading the participants' descriptions of the phenomenon to acquire a feeling for their experience and to make general sense of their experience
2. Extracting significant statements that pertain directly to the phenomenon under study
3. Formulating meanings for these significant statements to illuminate hidden meanings
4. Categorizing the meanings into clusters of themes and confirming consistency between the emerging findings and the participants' stories without giving in to the temptation to ignore data that do not "fit"

5. Integrating the findings into exhaustive description of the phenomenon under study; describing includes coding segments of text for topics, comparing topics for consistent themes, and bridging themes for their conceptual meanings, which leads to creating a prototype of a theoretical model about the phenomenon studied
6. Validating the findings by returning to the study participants to ask how the universal description compares with their personal experiences
7. Incorporating any changes offered by the participants into the final description of the phenomenon

Data analysis may also involve referring to the investigator's reflective journal and debriefing with experts on the phenomenological method and with persons who are not research participants but are familiar with the phenomenon.

Intuiting, the third strategy in descriptive phenomenological study, is attempting to gain an insight of what it might be like to "be in the study participants' shoes." As data are generated, the researcher's intuition is informed by attentive listening, self-reflection, and on going reflection regarding the commonalities across participants' stories. Intuiting balanced with bracketing involves a conscious attempt to honor the emerging evidence while refraining from prematurely foreclosing on the researcher's own biases or understandings (Wojnar & Swanson, 2007).

The culminating point of descriptive phenomenological investigation is to present a model representing the structure of the phenomenon under study (Colaizzi, 1978). Consistent with the Husserlian assumptions, if the true structure of the phenomenon is identified, then anyone who has experienced the phenomenon should be able to see their own experience in the proposed model or description.

DESCRIPTION OF THE STUDY

Our study started as an interdisciplinary community-based research project where a group of six faculty from our university were working with the neighborhood Head Start preschool. When engaging in community-based research, the research questions should come from the community partner; therefore, during the first 6 months of the project, we spent time exploring each other's histories, strengths, and resources. It was during this time that the Head Start staff became intrigued with Dr. Wojnar's phenomenological research project on the perinatal experiences of Somali couples, because the majority of the families enrolled in Head Start at that time were from Somalia. The staff asked us if it was possible to extend this research to investigate the Somali families' parenting of small children to ascertain whether their needs were being met by the Head Start program. It was the staff's impression there may have been gaps in their knowledge base about the particular needs of these families, particularly around culturally related expectations.

The internal review board (IRB) process was fairly quick, as we were able to build on the ethical approval Dr. Wojnar had previously submitted for her perinatal study with Somali parents by submitting modifications and requesting an extension. Once the IRB approval was obtained, our first task was to gain access to the Somali community served by the Head Start program. After meeting and strategizing with the Head Start staff, we were very fortunate to be put in contact with Mr. Abdisharid Issak, a Somali community caseworker and certified interpreter, who agreed to work with us. We didn't realize it initially, but our collaboration with Mr. Issak was a significant factor in opening doors into what is commonly known as a "difficult to reach" community. Through his work as a caseworker, Mr. Issak was not only acquainted with many of the families throughout the Seattle Somali community, but was also a well-respected and trusted member of the community. We made up flyers and posters to assist with recruitment of participants; however, it was Mr. Issak who did most of the recruiting for our study. Through grant funding, we were able to provide every family with a $50 Walmart gift card for participating in the study (Walmart was decided upon after consulting with the community representatives). Based on prior experience with conducting descriptive phenomenological research, our target sample was open ended (Wojnar & Swanson, 2007). After interviews with 20 families, the enrollment was closed, as no new conceptual information was emerging from the participants' stories (Wojnar & Swanson, 2007).

Collecting the Data

To begin our interviews, we met Mr. Issak at the Head Start main offices on a clear, cool October day. The Head Start office is located within the low-income housing unit neighborhood where many of the families served by the preschool reside. This particular housing community, Yesler Terrace, is part of the Seattle Housing Authority and has served low-income and refugee families since 1943. Yesler Terrace is comprised of about 500 housing units. Mr. Issak told us that he had enlisted a few families willing to participate in the study, and so we set off on foot for the first interview. We were amazed at how easily we were able to access families with Mr. Issak as our guide and recruiter.

Dr. Wojnar had also established a reputation as a trusted researcher from her previous experience within the Somali community. Initially, our questions focused on parent satisfaction with the services and programs provided by Head Start; however, one of the themes that emerged early on was that Somali parents revere teachers and consider them to be second parents in the family. Parents were therefore reluctant to criticize the Head Start staff in any way, but talked freely about their own challenges with parenting small children in the United States. Hence, after the first two interviews, we expanded our questions to explore challenges of parenting in the United States versus Somalia, and parents were eager to share. By the third interview, it was clear that parents also wanted to talk about hopes and dreams for their children in the United States, and so we added this topic to our dialogue.

Each interview was taped and later given to a transcriptionist to transcribe. During the interview, Dr. Bowie took detailed notes of parent answers, while Mr. Issak translated each question and answer for those who needed it. This procedure worked well, as it left Dr. Wojnar free to conduct the interviews.

Analyzing the Data

All transcripts were analyzed using the steps outlined by Colaizzi (1978), described in the preceding paragraphs. To aid credibility of findings, first each investigator coded the interviews separately and then met together to discuss and verify the information. Additionally, we used member check technique to validate the findings and consulted with Mr. Issak, our interpreter, to provide the contextual information that helped with the proper interpretation of data.

LESSONS LEARNED

Be Prepared to Adapt and Conduct the Research Differently Than You Planned

As mentioned previously, because of the cultural context and community needs, we shifted our broad research question somewhat after the first two interviews. In addition, we found that men shared more openly than women, which was a new experience to us as qualitative investigators. Often, the husband acted as spokesperson and interviewee for the family, and the wife would simply nod and agree with everything he said. We were careful not to press the women for their personal views, respecting this way of communication as a cultural norm.

We also learned very quickly that the trust of the dominant culture, in this case, us as researchers, can be an issue based on past experiences with various government, school, municipality officials, and others. There is also a possibility of shame for some within the community if one's individual opinions somehow were to be identified. For example, a few participants refused to be audiotaped for fear the taped interview could be lost and their voices identified. Moreover, one person did not want to sign the written consent form because of similar fears, although the same person did give oral consent to participate. After obtaining IRB approval to modify the original protocol, we included all of these individuals in the study, as they had equally important information to share. To this end, although the consent was verbally translated by the interpreter, it was our sense that the traditional IRB consent form, with all the information required to receive study approval, was intimidating, too detailed, and too complex for the parents we interviewed. If, in the future, we perform descriptive phenomenological research with a similar community, we will pursue crafting a more culturally appropriate consent form with the help of the community representative and explain this approach to the IRB members in the initial submission.

Test the Recording Equipment Prior to Each Interview and Expect the Unexpected

It was not uncommon, particularly in Somali Bantu households, for there to be no Western-type furniture such as tables and chairs. In these instances, we usually sat on thick Persian-type rugs and had to place our recorder on the floor, which created a challenge to acquiring quality sound recordings. Moreover, many houses were full of young children, who can be noisy, and parts of some of the interviews were very difficult for the transcriptionist to understand. Dr. Bowie's notes were then invaluable in filling in holes; however, she could not be present at every interview, so some of the transcriptions had gaps. We also recommend placing any recording equipment as close to the interpreter as possible. In hindsight, it would have been helpful to use a microphone for the interpreter rather than place the recorder on a table or floor midway between the study participants and interpreter. For example, the voice that we needed to hear most clearly on the recording was that of the interpreter, but it seemed more natural to place the recorder next to the client.

Be Aware of the Changing Stakeholders Within the Community

We had reached out to the community through our primary community partner, Head Start; however, midway through the interviews, informal leadership within the community shifted when a Somali woman from another area assumed an important position within the Yesler Terrace Housing Authority. Initially, we were not aware of this woman's formal position and the informal power she held within the community, and we also did not realize that she was concerned about the university faculty team conducting research with members of the Somali community. When we (accidentally) found out about her concerns, we immediately set up meetings with her to discuss the project and our intentions as researchers within the community. However, it was a difficult, if not impossible, task to establish trust with this community leader after the research project was already underway. During this process, we realized how important it is to be aware of changing community leadership, identifying possible trigger points, and responding promptly to direct and indirect verbal and nonverbal cues from the stakeholders. In hindsight, we realize we should have been more visible at community meetings and school events. Our entire faculty team made a concerted effort to interface with the Yesler Terrace community on a regular basis, but a more purposeful plan may have helped decrease or prevent the concerns of the new community leader.

Uncovering the Cultural Context

There are many layers to uncover in understanding the cultural context using a phenomenological approach. As previously described, researchers' own prejudicial views, preunderstandings, biases, and experiences need to be openly faced and set aside throughout the research process. Identifying the cultural norms of the population studied is also central to this process. For example, Somali families are typically large, as children are viewed as gifts from God; the largest families are commonly considered the wealthiest and most blessed. In Somalia, children are free to roam, and parenting is a shared responsibility among extended family and all members of the community. We heard from several families how fearful they were of Child Protective Services (CPS) taking their children away, as they had heard horror stories from other Somali families who, unknowingly, allowed their children to roam the neighborhoods when first moving to the United States. Stories like this affirmed the closeness of this community and how quickly word can travel throughout.

Previously, we mentioned the Somali parents' high regard for their children's teachers. Somali parents defer to teachers as the experts and do not understand the Western value of parental partnering with teachers for decision making around the educational needs of children and helping with homework or school projects. In fact, the majority of research participants had no educational preparation or knowledge of the English language to meet the expectation of helping their children with schoolwork. It was important for us to understand this view, as it partly explained why Somali parents were sometimes confused about the Western expectation to actively participate in their child's education by volunteering in the classroom and ensuring that homework is completed. It also clarified for us why Somali parents did not have an opinion about the types of programs that should be offered to their children, as they viewed the teachers as the experts in determining their children's educational needs.

Finally, one should give consideration to the stages of integration into a new culture and country for a refugee population as an essential piece of understanding the lived experience. Ager and Strang (2008) identify core domains of integration, including but not limited to housing, employment, education, and health. Obtaining paid employment is an essential step to integrating into a new home country, yet with minimal or no formal education, finding work is difficult for many Somalis. We met several Somali women who had opened in-home day care centers to provide sources of income for their families. While this work is resourceful, it can put a strain on families whose cultural norm is a patriarchal model that traces ancestry through their fathers (Boyle & Ali, 2009). Within the Somali culture, men traditionally make family decisions and work outside the home and women raise the children and care for the home. When Somali mothers are working, it may be more difficult for the family to integrate as smoothly into other important domains of society such as the educational system. Recognizing these stages of integration can assist qualitative researchers working with recent immigrants to formulate questions that delve into issues that are the most critical for the community members.

SUMMARY

In summary, using a phenomenological research approach to gather information about a specific community's lived experience can not only be helpful in gaining a better understanding of that community's cultural context, but can also assist in the design of programs that are most relevant for that particular community. We have emphasized the importance of putting aside preconceived ideas about the community under investigation when using this research approach, yet it is also necessary to have some understanding of the culture to avoid embarking upon interviews that may offend or alienate members of the community. It is a difficult balancing act, particularly when working with a vulnerable refugee population who may have experienced the stresses of war, poverty, and life in refugee camps. Identifying and establishing working relationships with trusted leaders of the community is, therefore, an essential piece of using the phenomenological research method within community-based research.

REFERENCES

Ager, A., & Strang, A. (2008). Understanding integration: A conceptual framework. *Journal of Refugee Studies, 21*(2), 166–191.

Boyle, E. H., & Ali, A. (2009). Culture, structure, and the refugee experience in Somali immigrant family transformation. *International Migration, 48*(1), 47–49. doi:10.1111/j.1468-2435.2009.00512.x

Colaizzi, P. F. (1978). Psychological research as the phenomenologist views it. In R. Valle & M. King (Eds.), *Existential phenomenological alternatives for psychology* (pp. 48–71). New York, NY: Oxford University Press.

Deutscher, M. (2001). Husserl's transcendental subjectivity. In R. Small (Ed.), *A hundred years of phenomenology. Perspectives on a philosophical tradition* (pp. 3–25). Burlington, VT: Ashgate Publishing.

Giorgi, A. (2000). The status of Husserlian phenomenology in caring research. *Scandinavian Journal of Caring Sciences, 14*(1), 3–10.

Husserl, E. (1970). *Logical investigations* (J. N. Findlay, Trans.). New York, NY: Humanities Press.

Husserl, E. (2001). *Analyses concerning passive and active synthesis: Lectures on transcendental logic* (A. J. Steinbeck, Trans.). Boston, MA: Kluwer Academic Publishers.

LeVasseur, J. J. (2003). The problem of bracketing in phenomenology. *Qualitative Health Research, 13*(3), 408–420.

Lopez, K. A., & Willis, D. G. (2004). Descriptive versus interpretive phenomenology: Their contributions to nursing knowledge. *Qualitative Health Research, 14*(5), 726–735.

Moran, D. (2000). *Introduction to phenomenology.* London, UK: Routledge.

Swanson, K. M., & Wojnar, D. (2004). Optimal healing environments in nursing. *Journal of Alternative and Complementary Medicine, 10*, S43–S48.

Swanson-Kauffman, K. M. (1986). Caring in the instance of unexpected early pregnancy loss. *Topics in Clinical Nursing, 8*(2), 37–46.

Swanson-Kauffman, K. M., & Schonwald, E. (1988). Phenomenology. In B. Sarter (Ed.), *Paths to knowledge: Innovative research methods for nursing* (pp. 97–105). New York, NY: National League for Nursing.

Tymieniecka, M. T. (2003). Introduction: Phenomenology as the inspirational force of our times. In M. T. Tymieniecka (Ed.), *Phenomenology world-wide. Foundations—expanding dynamics—life-engagements. A guide for research and study* (pp. 1–10). London, UK: Kluwer Academic Publishers.

Wall, C., Glenn, S., Mitchinson, S., & Poole, H. (2004). Using reflective diary to develop bracketing skills during a phenomenological investigation. *Nurse Researcher, 11*(4), 20–29.

Wojnar, D. M., & Swanson, K. M. (2007). Phenomenology: An exploration. *Journal of Holistic Nursing, 25*(3), 172–180.

CHAPTER EIGHT

BEING THE PARENT OF AN INFANT WITH COLIC: A PHENOMENOLOGICAL HERMENEUTIC PERSPECTIVE

Kajsa Landgren

Over the past few decades, I have had the opportunity to meet many parents of infants with colic. After hearing their stories, I decided to conduct a qualitative study in the hopes of giving them a voice. My supervisor and I interpreted interviews together with a phenomenological hermeneutic method described by Lindseth and Norberg (2004). The results of the study were published in the article "Parents' experience of living with a baby with infantile colic—A phenomenological hermeneutic study" (Landgren & Hallström, 2011).

DESCRIPTION OF THE STUDY

We designed the study as a qualitative and inductive study wherein mothers and fathers were interviewed about their experiences of having a baby with infantile colic; and we interviewed them in the middle of the colicky period. Our objective was to shed light on the meaning of this phenomenon. The main theme that emerged was "Colic overshadows everything" with the subthemes "Living in an inferno," "Missing the situation dreamt of," and "Surviving infantile colic." In the families who shared their experiences, it was not only the infants who were affected by colic. Parents suffered with their babies and felt hopeless, as they could not comfort their child, which they perceived as their main task in life. Unable to stop their babies' cries, parents became overwhelmed by strong feelings such as frustration, helplessness, guilt, and shame. They worried constantly, feeling exhausted and worn out as they tried every possible strategy to comfort their babies.

Intrafamily relations were challenged; sharing the burden with someone became critically important. Most parents shared this with their partners, and those who could not shared with other adults such as nurses or their own parents.

RELEVANCE TO NURSING

Sickness and suffering are personal experiences and can have a meaning. According to Travelbee, "standing in the patient's shoes" can shift nurses' perspective, leading to greater understanding and empathy, which are essential to nursing (Travelbee, 1971). In my example of infantile colic, the nurse has a role not only in aiding the suffering infants by helping parents find interventions that soothe the infants' pain, but also in helping parents to maintain hope, to cope with the stress and suffering, to endure and handle the situation, and to find a meaning in the experience; this is one of the nurses' most important tasks. It is the nurse's responsibility to help create a context in which this is possible, using herself as a therapeutic tool (Travelbee, 1971). If parents lose hope, it will affect the important parent–child bond. For professional interaction, nurses must understand their patients' perspectives. As our outlook on phenomena changes, our behavior also changes. Hopefully, this study will make it easier for nurses to understand parents' life worlds, to sympathize with them, and to develop a therapeutic alliance. If readers of phenomenological research integrate their interpretation into their worlds, they can be more productive in life and in clinical work.

METHODOLOGY

Researchers generally look for a method well suited to their research question. In this case, I wanted to shed light on and interpret parents' experiences in the way that they themselves described it, to elucidate, unfold, and uncover the essential meaning of their lived experiences. Both phenomenology and hermeneutics can be useful when applied to existential questions with more than one answer or interpretation. Phenomenology includes a variety of methods, all aiming to analyze stories about the lived experience to reveal the essential meaning of a phenomenon. When I studied qualitative research, I perceived pure phenomenology as leading to a result that was too abstract to be useful. One of the exercises in my phenomenology course was to describe a phenomenon together with some course participants and then to ask willing passersby to identify it. During the second part of the exercise, it became obvious that other people could not recognize the described phenomenon. Then and there, I realized that I could not handle the abstractness of traditional phenomenology.

Hermeneutics, on the other hand, concerns understanding through interpretation. In reference to Heidegger, Mackey states that "[w]hen things in the world have been understood through interpretation we can say that they have a meaning" (Mackey, 2005, p. 182). Natural science is inadequate for understanding human beings. To interpret information is to render it understandable, to make complex and layered impressions comprehensible. The interpretation itself is subjective and selective, and the individual interprets according to personal expectations, wishes, and previous experiences. More or less knowingly, people always use interpretations to orient themselves in the world. Within hermeneutics, these interpretations are emphasized. As we are interpretive beings, we have already interpreted the phenomenon according to the cultures to which we belong. The phenomenon is hidden—it already exists but needs visibility. In other words, interpretation is disclosure of what is already there.

However, a blended version of phenomenology and hermeneutics attracted me most. We chose the phenomenological hermeneutic method described by Lindseth and Norberg (2004), which aims to elucidate the essential meaning in the lived experience as understood by the interpreter, thereby making it possible to see our world with a new perspective. We did not expect to find a unique fundamental truth because the whole truth can never be fully understood. However, this type of research is a way to seek out possible meanings in a continuous process. The method allows a personal, colorful writing style, where you can take the patients' part and give them a voice. The method is inspired by philosopher Paul Ricoeur, who presented the idea of this combined method of describing and interpreting.

In phenomenological hermeneutics, the starting point is the text produced from narrative interviews. Listening to others' narratives and narrating our own experiences is a basic way to gain understanding. The stories shed light on lived experiences and the possibilities of living in the world and reveal the essential meaning of the studied phenomena. The goal is to understand the experiences of good and bad expressed in the interviews. It is not the text itself but the ethics expressed therein that should be investigated. The text should be interpreted without judging its correctness. Retelling an event brings the past into the present and influences the future. In our study, we wanted to give parents of infants with colic the opportunity to talk about their life world, about their being in the world, and thereby help us understand what it means to have a baby that you cannot comfort. Through their narratives, we can participate in their world, understand the experiences expressed in the interviews, and comprehend the structure of their lived experiences in a way that enables us to grasp the nature and significance of this experience.

Of course, another factor in my decision was chance. When I was planning the study, I had an opportunity to take part in two courses. The first was a course in phenomenological writing with Fredricka Gilje (University of Alaska Anchorage, Anchorage, Alaska) and Ingegerd Fagerberg (Mälardalens Högskola, Sweden), both enthusiastic experts in phenomenology. The second was a course in the application of phenomenological hermeneutics led by Astrid Norberg (Umeå University, Sweden), who, together with Anders Lindseth (Tromsö University, Norway), authored the article outlining how to apply the method (Lindseth & Norberg, 2004). Both courses were deeply inspiring. As I was a novice in the different qualitative methods, I would be remiss if I failed to acknowledge the possibility of these two courses having affected my decision. Taking the courses while analyzing the data provided a great opportunity. The guidance in phenomenological writing inspired me at just the right moment, and I could use parts of my own interviews as examples for course exercises, which were supervised by one of the method's founders.

Sample

We included 23 parents (12 mothers and 11 fathers, representing 14 families). We did not encounter the usual difficulty of recruiting enough participants—all but two who were asked to participate agreed. The interviews were long, emotional, and detailed, lending a rare richness and depth to the data.

One condition for quality in phenomenological hermeneutic analyses is good narrative interviews (Lindseth & Norberg, 2004). Researchers have spent too much time analyzing poor interviews (Norberg, personal communication, 2006). Even if a good analysis can save a less fruitful interview text, the importance of conducting good interviews cannot be overemphasized. The informants must be appropriate for the research question and willing and able to tell their stories. So, one must choose participants based on those criteria. Therefore, in this study, I chose parents who were in the middle of the colicky period. To obtain different perspectives, we chose both mothers and fathers, first-time parents, those who had had children before, older and younger parents, and so on. All informants were eager to tell their stories except for one father who did not understand why I wanted him to tell his story, as he felt it was not his job to take care of the baby. However, he accepted the invitation to participate. Though this interview was shorter than the other interviews, it still provided valuable information about the different life worlds of the parents of babies with colic. This interview illustrated the range of approaches to parenting, whereas the others added more depth and shed light on a particular approach.

I continued to interview as I began writing the transcription and analysis. If I had analyzed each interview before conducting the next one, I could have stopped earlier, as the last interviews revealed no new findings. Having more informants and interviews than needed for saturation is time consuming, and handling more text than necessary is impractical. However, I felt surer of the validity of the results. In future studies, I will follow the advice from Kvale (1994, p. 165): "Interview so many subjects that you find out what you need to know."

If I could have done anything differently, I would have tried harder to find a single mother. In the article, many mothers felt that they had no one with whom to share their experience, but none of them actually lived alone with the crying baby. Furthermore, several of the infants in this sample were born prematurely, leading to some uncertainty as to whether I had studied colic or prematurity. This recruitment bias arose due to an overlap with the recruitment period for another trial including infants with colic. In that trial, which also evaluated the effect of acupuncture, prematurity was an exclusion criterion. We considered being interviewed to be an intervention, as telling your story can change your perception, so no babies were allowed to take part in both studies. Unfortunately, this resulted in more premature babies in the interview study.

Ethical Considerations

Ethical approval was obtained from Lund University's Research Ethics Committee. The participants were in a vulnerable situation but agreed to share their stories, providing written informed consent after receiving written information about the study. They were informed that it would not be possible to identify the participating families. Any clues, such as their towns, their hospitals, and their family members' names were coded; and quotes were marked "M4" for "mother number 4." After the interview, some mentioned how much of a relief it had been to talk about their experiences.

Setting

Parents chose the dates and locations for the interviews. All but one couple chose to be interviewed in their homes, where it was easier for them to relax. If the other parent was present, that person took care of the baby during the interview, but they were not allowed to listen or to participate. To avoid the partner's influence, I conducted interviews individually. After the first parent was interviewed, he or she took over caring for the baby if the second parent had agreed to participate. As I was a guest in their home, I did as I was invited to do and tried to make them feel as safe and as comfortable as possible. I did not wear a nurse uniform. If the parents offered coffee, I politely declined, as drinking coffee might prove distracting for me during the interview. However, I made it clear that they themselves were welcome to do so if it made them feel more relaxed.

Taking care of a baby, especially one with colic, can make it difficult to adhere to a time limit. I ensured that I had plenty of time so that stress would not lower the quality of the interviews. Additionally, this allowed the informants to form and expand their thoughts. If the baby cried or needed feeding, we paused the interview momentarily while the baby and the parent settled down. Interviewing in their homes also gave me a wider perspective and allowed me to better understand their situation.

Rigor

To achieve trustworthiness, we followed the steps described by Lindseth and Norberg (2004). The first naive interpretation, which was a guess, was followed by a very structured analysis of all collected data. I was a doctoral student and performed the analysis in close cooperation with my co-author and supervisor professor Inger Hallström (Lund University, Sweden). We analyzed the interviews separately at first (intercoder reliability) and then comparatively. I categorized the same interview twice and found the same themes (intracoder reliability). I am aware that the result can differ with longer intervals between analyses, even with the same researcher, but in this case, the result of the second analysis was very close to that of the first.

Following Lindseth and Norberg's instructions (Lindseth & Norberg, 2004), we entered the hermeneutic circle by moving through the three methodological steps: naive reading, structural analysis, and comprehensive understanding. This seemed hopelessly theoretical to me before I began analyzing, so it was surprising to experience the dialectic movement between understanding and explanation as it began to take shape. This process between interpretation and understanding, between the parts and the whole, went back and forth until the naive interpretation and the themes matched up. By then, I knew the text so well that I could hear the informants' voices upon re-reading it. The analyses took time—almost a year, in fact. However, I did not need to rush. The data were thoroughly processed, which allowed time for the themes and subthemes to emerge from the text in an honest way inclusive of all details. In the final portion of this step, the findings were validated with the existing literature.

Of course, transferability relies on being able to analyze the context, so we described the informants in terms of gender, age, living condition, and family situation.

The findings were presented and discussed at seminars with nursing colleagues and midwives in our research group. They gave valuable comments and confirmed the findings. For example, one of the subthemes, *Feeling hope, happiness, and gratitude*, was formulated after such a meeting. One colleague found the presented result to be negative and asked if no one expressed hope. I went back to the text, found a few meaning units expressing those positive sentiments, and so added that theme.

The phenomenological hermeneutic method requires high-quality narrative interviews. Informants must know the phenomenon and be willing and able to speak about their experiences. Naturally, in the present study, participants were well aware of the phenomenon of having a baby with colic—they were living in colicky chaos! They spoke openly and at length, baring their emotions, even crying at times. The narratives were rich in depth as well as in breadth, and thus were capable of providing the basis for a trustworthy analysis.

We used quotes from the interviews to confirm the result further. It was difficult to choose from the many valuable quotes found in the 220 single-spaced pages of transcribed interviews. I felt responsible for conveying the parents' experiences—omitting information felt like omitting a voice. I found it a bit painful to exclude some magnificent quotes to reduce the text to a publishable size.

It is sometimes said that researchers should bracket their preunderstanding, but this is a difficult, if not impossible, task. Instead, we made our preunderstandings visible by describing how I originally met the families included in the study—initially as a nurse at a pediatric emergency unit and then for 10 years at an acupuncture clinic—and how my supervisor had extensive experience involving work and research on infants and parents. In the article, we described preunderstanding as a part of the interpretative process and as a guiding tool. It is often stated in qualitative articles that the authors discuss and reflect on their preunderstandings, but we opted to approach this more organically, discussing any doubts about our interpretations as they arose.

Four years later, we conducted follow-up interviews with the same parents to investigate the aftereffects of the colicky period (Landgren, Lundqvist, & Hallström, 2012). By that time, we had a major preunderstanding of the parents' life worlds. As the phenomenological hermeneutic method is more suitable to inductive research, we chose content analysis for the follow-up interviews.

It is a challenge to bridle the impulse to overinterpret, but I was so concerned about it that I may have underinterpreted instead. For example, several parents expressed how acupuncture had helped their older children with colic. As I am also an acupuncturist, I wanted to avoid any accusations of bias and so only mentioned these comments in a few sentences.

DATA COLLECTION AND ANALYSIS PROCEDURES

In this study, the parents were encouraged to narrate their experiences of having a baby with colic, to give their version of the phenomenon, and to share their life world. They were asked open-ended questions that prompted reflection. I conducted all interviews and followed an interview guide, meaning that I started with the question: "Can you tell me about your experiences of having an infant with colic?" Most informants were very talkative. If they stopped talking or lost their train of thought, and/or if I wanted to check my understanding, I asked follow-up questions aimed at encouraging further narration, such as: "How did you feel then?" or "Can you describe it another way?"

However, not everyone is a born interviewer! Conducting good interviews is a hard-earned skill. When I listened to the tape recordings from my first interviews, I felt embarrassed. I could hear myself almost interrupting informants in my eagerness to understand everything correctly. With repeated practice came more awareness, and I learned not to be afraid of silence, to allow informants more time to reflect and space to speak.

The parents determined the lengths of their interviews, which lasted between 17 and 55 minutes (median 35 minutes). Directly after each interview, I made a summary of the information so that the participant could comment and reflect on his/her narrative. Even this part of the interview was tape-recorded. I took some field notes during the interview to help me remember things not represented in the audio recording, such as movements or nonverbal reactions.

Conducting the interviews took a year (2006–2007), and the analysis and article writing took an additional year of intense work. All interviews were transcribed verbatim by me, and those many hours of transcribing allowed, and sometimes forced, me to come closer to the text. Letting a secretary perform this task would have saved much time, but I am glad I had to listen to the interviews over and over again while I was writing. The text was punctuated to reflect the informants' meanings. Pauses and nonverbal expressions were noted, which was helpful later on. For example, the text could read "... when he is crying ... *pauses 5 seconds* ... *sighs heavy* ... *pauses another 10 seconds* ... it makes me feel so ... so ... so helpless." While doing analyzing, the punctuation helped me remember the participants' difficulties with formulating a certain experience and how they narrated their stories.

To understand and interpret the text, we went through the three methodological steps of phenomenological hermeneutic analysis. During the naive reading, my co-author and I read the text several times to grasp its meaning as a whole, and we tried to be open to whatever the text communicated. A researcher cannot be neutral. The text can "attack you," and that can be painful. We allowed ourselves to feel touched and moved by it. Then, we tried to switch from a natural attitude to a phenomenological attitude and formulated the naive understanding as a metaphor: The parents were tired passengers on a stormy sea. Having lost control, they were terrified of drowning, but no one could help them. Suffering with their baby, clinging to each other for help, they searched for survival strategies.

The next step was a thematic structural analysis to validate the naive understanding, resulting in finding themes conveying the essential meaning of the parents' lived experiences. The text was divided into meaning units and entered into a table. A meaning unit could be a few words or several sentences. Too small meaning units give unwanted fragmentation, while too big meaning units might cause us to overlook something substantial. If upon further analysis, a meaning unit appeared to encompass multiple codes, it was then divided as such. To make it easier to find usable quotes, I highlighted potential meaning units while processing the text in the table.

The meaning units were condensed and abstracted in the table so that the essential meaning of each meaning unit was expressed with everyday words. We then read and reflected upon all codes, seeking out similarities and differences. Similar condensed meanings formed subthemes, which we assembled into themes, and, finally, a main theme took shape.

The themes were compared and reflected upon in relation to the naive understanding for validation. I began the analysis with each interview in a separate file. When the themes took shape, I created a separate file for each one to gain a better overview. I checked and discussed the themes with my co-author until we achieved consensus. The analysis was performed repeatedly until the naive understanding and the themes matched each other and the themes validated the naive understanding.

Finally, we reflected upon the naive understanding and the themes in relation to relevant books and articles about the meaning of the lived experience. This part of the writing process—the comprehensive understanding—is essential, according to Ricoeur, and can disclose new possibilities for being in the world. You are supposed to use your imagination and relevant literature to revise and deepen your understanding of the text. This was the most difficult part of the analysis, as it was tricky to find adequate articles to illustrate the connection between theory and phenomenon. The reviewers of the first journal to which I submitted the script did not recognize my suggested references on systems theory and a model of family-focused nursing as nursing theories. My unwillingness to let go of these theories led to a refusal—which delayed publication for almost a year—and a note to self: Never question a reviewer's idea of which theories are valid.

The results were formulated in everyday language as close to lived experience as possible. Following the parents' example, we did not avoid strong diction, e.g. chaos or inferno, in our attempt to evoke a sense of their experiences in the reader. Verbs, rather than nouns, were used to describe their lived experience. We used gerunds to convey immediacy and urgency (e.g., being, feeling). Metaphors and similes were used to convey the interpreted meanings. Everything said, unsaid, or expressed in other ways can be subject to interpretation. I tried to shed light on the patterns as well as on the phenomena that did not follow them. Analyzing these phenomena—for example, a mother of colicky twins claiming to be grateful, proud, and hopeful—can increase validity, because it provides a wider range of perspectives.

CHALLENGES

I had to remind myself often that my results described the life worlds of real people, who, in my case, were 23 parents with colicky infants. The result was a description of their life worlds, though these are not the only possible ones. It can be tempting to assume that the result mirrors the situation for all people in similar circumstances. Likewise, it can be hard to refrain from drawing conclusions about cause and effect (Paley, 2005).

Furthermore, the interviewer and the informant affect each other, so the interviewer is definitely involved in producing the narrative that becomes the data used for the analyses. I found it can be a challenge to stay neutral when interviewing and not reveal your own opinions. My duty was to take the participants' perspective without judging, even if I didn't sympathize with them. In this study, I could easily sympathize with the parents, but in some cases, I felt a slight irritation when I thought informants had unrealistic or overly romantic expectations of parenthood; in one particular interview, I was upset by a father who stated that the baby's crying was not his responsibility. In these interviews, I had to concentrate on not indicating my viewpoint, and I got to practice confirming their emotions without supporting their opinions. It became obvious for me that understanding informants' life worlds could lead to sympathy and that each interview replenished my inner reference system, making it easier for me to better understand other informants.

Another challenge was to think phenomenologically initially before transitioning to hermeneutic reflection, constantly moving in the hermeneutic spiral between the parts and the whole without losing perspective. On the one hand, I had to be open and responsive, allowing myself to be affected and surprised. On the other hand, I had to distance myself, which felt confusing at times. It can take a while to balance the daring required to interpret the latent meaning with the fear of overinterpreting. I could not afford to take anything for granted. I had to look at the themes as they came up without preconceptions, and I could not assume that I knew what the informants were going to say (and therefore only hear select parts of their stories). Additionally, I needed to listen to what they left unsaid and reflect on why because, at times, those details proved vital.

Heidegger states that "only the leap into the river tells us what is called swimming" (Hultgren, 1995). True enough, I only learned phenomenology through practice. I realized that, sometimes, you just have to get started, that you and your skills will develop organically during the process (Hultgren, 1995).

Of course, qualitative research is deeply time consuming, and in a scientific community imbued with quantitative standards, it can be a challenge to communicate the necessity of understanding the meaning of someone's lived experience. However, in continuously applying for grants, we can push for more qualitative studies, which are essential to nursing research.

REFERENCES

Hultgren, F. (1995). The phenomenology of "doing" phenomenology: The experience of teaching and learning together. *Human Studies, 18*, 371–388.

Kvale, S. (1994). Ten standard objections to qualitative research interviews. *Journal of Phenomenological Psychology, 25*(2), 147–173.

Landgren, K., & Hallstrom, I. (2011). Parents' experience of living with a baby with infantile colic—A phenomenological hermeneutic study. *Scandinavian Journal of Caring Science, 25*(2), 317–324.

Landgren, K., Lundqvist, A., & Hallström, I. (2012). Remembering the chaos—But life went on and the wound healed. A four year follow up with parents having had a baby with infantile colic. *The Open Nursing Journal, 6,* 48–56.

Lindseth, A., & Norberg, A. (2004). A phenomenological hermeneutical method for researching lived experience. *Scandinavian Journal of Caring Science, 18,* 145–153.

Mackey, S. (2005). Phenomenological nursing research: Methodological insights derived from Heidegger's interpretive phenomenology. *International Journal of Nursing Studies, 42,* 179–186.

Paley, J. (2005). Phenomenology as rhetoric. *Nursing Inquiry, 12*(2), 106–116.

Travelbee, J. (1971). *Interpersonal aspects of nursing* (2nd ed.). Philadelphia, PA: F. A. Davis.

LIST OF JOURNALS THAT PUBLISH QUALITATIVE RESEARCH

Mary de Chesnay

Conducting excellent research and not publishing the results negates the study and prohibits anyone from learning from the work. Therefore, it is critical that qualitative researchers disseminate their work widely, and the best way to do so is through publication in refereed journals. The peer review process, although seemingly brutal at times, is designed to improve knowledge by enhancing the quality of literature in a discipline. Fortunately, the publishing climate has evolved to the point where qualitative research is valued by editors and readers alike, and many journals now seek out, or even specialize in publishing, qualitative research.

The following table was compiled partially from the synopsis of previous work identifying qualitative journals by the St. Louis University Qualitative Research Committee (2013), with a multidisciplinary faculty, who are proponents of qualitative research. Many of these journals would be considered multidisciplinary, though marketed to nurses. All are peer reviewed. Other journals were identified by the author of this series and by McKibbon and Gadd (2004) in their quantitative analysis of qualitative research. It is not meant to be exhaustive, and we would welcome any suggestions for inclusion.

An additional resource is the nursing literature mapping project conducted by Sherwill-Navarro and Allen (Allen, Jacobs, & Levy, 2006). The 217 journals were listed as a resource for libraries to accrue relevant journals, and many of them publish qualitative research. Readers are encouraged to view the websites for specific journals that might be interested in publishing their studies. Readers are also encouraged to look outside the traditional nursing journals, especially if their topics more closely match the journal mission of related disciplines.

NURSING JOURNALS

Journal	Website
Advances in Nursing Science	www.journals.lww.com/advancesinnursingscience/pages/default.aspx
Africa Journal of Nursing and Midwifery	www.journals.co.za/ej/ejour_ajnm.html
Annual Review of Nursing Research	www.springerpub.com/product/07396686#.UeaXbjvvv6U
British Journal of Nursing	www.britishjournalofnursing.com
Canadian Journal of Nursing Research	www.cjnr.mcgill.ca
Hispanic Health Care International	www.springerpub.com/product/15404153#.UeaX7jvvv6U
Holistic Nursing Practice	www.journals.lww.com/hnpjournal/pages/default.aspx
International Journal of Mental Health Nursing	www.onlinelibrary.wiley.com/journal/10.1111/(ISSN)1447-0349
International Journal of Nursing Practice	www.onlinelibrary.wiley.com/journal/10.1111/(ISSN)1440-172X
International Journal of Nursing Studies	www.journals.elsevier.com/international-journal-of-nursing-studies
Journal of Advanced Nursing	www.onlinelibrary.wiley.com/journal/10.1111/(ISSN)1365-2648
Journal of Clinical Nursing	www.onlinelibrary.wiley.com/journal/10.1111/(ISSN)1365-2702
Journal of Family Nursing	www.jfn.sagepub.com
Journal of Nursing Education	www.healio.com/journals/JNE
Journal of Nursing Scholarship	www.onlinelibrary.wiley.com/journal/10.1111/(ISSN)1547-5069
Nurse Researcher	www.nurseresearcher.rcnpublishing.co.uk
Nursing History Review	www.aahn.org/nhr.html
Nursing Inquiry	www.onlinelibrary.wiley.com/journal/10.1111/(ISSN)1440-1800
Nursing Research	www.ninr.nih.gov
Nursing Science Quarterly	www.nsq.sagepub.com
Online Brazilian Journal of Nursing	www.objnursing.uff.br/index.php/nursing

(continued)

Journal	Website
The Online Journal of Cultural Competence in Nursing and Healthcare	www.ojccnh.org
Public Health Nursing	www.onlinelibrary.wiley.com/journal/10.1111 /(ISSN)1525-1446
Qualitative Health Research	www.qhr.sagepub.com
Qualitative Research in Nursing and Healthcare	www.wiley.com/WileyCDA/WileyTitle/product Cd-1405161221.html
Research and Theory for Nursing Practice	www.springerpub.com/product/15416577#.Ueab lTvvv6U
Scandinavian Journal of Caring Sciences	www.onlinelibrary.wiley.com/journal/10.1111 /(ISSN)1471-6712
Western Journal of Nursing Research	http://wjn.sagepub.com

REFERENCES

Allen, M., Jacobs, S. K., & Levy, J. R. (2006). Mapping the literature of nursing: 1996–2000. *Journal of the Medical Library Association, 94*(2), 206–220. Retrieved from http://nahrs.mlanet.org/home/images/activity/nahrs2012selectedlist nursing.pdf

McKibbon, K., & Gadd, C. (2004). A quantitative analysis of qualitative studies in clinical journals for the publishing year 2000. *BMC Med Inform Decision Making, 4*, 11. Retrieved from http://www.ncbi.nlm.nih.gov/pmc/articles/PMC503397

St. Louis University Qualitative Research Committee. Retrieved July 14, 2013, from http://www.slu.edu/organizations/qrc/QRjournals.html

ESSENTIAL ELEMENTS FOR A QUALITATIVE PROPOSAL

Tommie Nelms

1. Introduction: Aim of the study
   a. Phenomenon of interest and focus of inquiry
   b. Justification for studying the phenomenon (how big an issue/problem?)
   c. Phenomenon discussed within a specific context (lived experience, culture, human response)
   d. Theoretical framework(s)
   e. Assumptions, biases, experiences, intuitions, and perceptions related to the belief that inquiry into a phenomenon is important (researcher's relationship to the topic)
   f. Qualitative methodology chosen, with rationale
   g. Significance to nursing (How will the new knowledge gained benefit patients, nursing practice, nurses, society, etc.?)
      Note: The focus of interest/inquiry and statement of purpose of the study should appear at the top of page 3 of the proposal
2. Literature review: What is known about the topic? How has it been studied in the past?
   Include background of the theoretical framework and how it has been used in the past.
3. Methodology
   a. Introduction of methodology (philosophical underpinnings of the method)
   b. Rationale for choosing the methodology
   c. Background of methodology
   d. Outcome of methodology
   e. Methods: general sources, and steps and procedures
   f. Translation of concepts and terms

4. Methods
   a. Aim
   b. Participants
   c. Setting
   d. Gaining access, and recruitment of participants
   e. General steps in conduct of study (data gathering tool(s), procedures, etc.)
   f. Human subjects' considerations
   g. Expected timetable
   h. Framework for rigor, and specific strategies to ensure rigor
   i. Plans and procedures for data analysis

WRITING QUALITATIVE RESEARCH PROPOSALS

Joan L. Bottorff

PURPOSE OF A RESEARCH PROPOSAL

- Communicates research plan to others (e.g., funding agencies)
- Serves as a detailed plan of action
- Serves as a contract between investigator and funding bodies when proposal is approved

QUALITATIVE RESEARCH: BASIC ASSUMPTIONS

- Reality is complex, constructed, and, ultimately, subjective.
- Research is an interpretative process.
- Knowledge is best achieved by conducting research in the natural setting.

QUALITATIVE RESEARCH

- Qualitative research is unstructured.
- Qualitative designs are "emergent" rather than fixed.
- The results of qualitative research are unpredictable (Morse, 1994).

KINDS OF QUALITATIVE RESEARCH

- Grounded theory
- Ethnography (critical ethnography, institutional ethnography, ethno-methodology, ethnoscience, etc.)
- Phenomenology
- Narrative inquiry
- Others

CHALLENGES FOR QUALITATIVE RESEARCHERS

- Developing a solid, convincing argument that the study contributes to theory, research, practice, and/or policy (the "so what?" question)
- Planning a study that is systematic, manageable, and flexible (to reassure skeptics):
  - Justification of the selected qualitative method
  - Explicit details about design and methods, without limiting the project's evolution
  - Attention to criteria for the overall soundness or rigor of the project

QUESTIONS A PROPOSAL MUST ANSWER

- Why should anyone be interested in my research?
- Is the research design credible, achievable, and carefully explained?
- Is the researcher capable of conducting the research? (Marshall & Rossman, 1999)

TIPS TO ANSWER THESE QUESTIONS

- Be practical (practical problems cannot be easily brushed off)
- Be persuasive ("sell" your proposal)
- Make broad links (hint at the wider context)
- Aim for crystal clarity (avoid jargon, assume nothing, explain everything) (Silverman, 2000)

SECTIONS OF A TYPICAL QUALITATIVE PROPOSAL

- Introduction
  - Introduction of topic and its significance
  - Statement of purpose, research questions/objectives
- Review of literature
  - Related literature and theoretical traditions
- Design and methods
  - Overall approach and rationale
  - Sampling, data gathering methods, data analysis
  - Trustworthiness (soundness of the research)
  - Ethical considerations
- Dissemination and knowledge translation
  - Timeline
  - Budget
  - Appendices

INTRODUCING THE STUDY—FIRST PARA

- Goal: Capture interest in the study
  - Focus on the importance of the study (Why bother with the question?)
  - Be clear and concise (details will follow)
  - Provide a synopsis of the primary target of the study
  - Present persuasive logic backed up with factual evidence

THE PROBLEM/RESEARCH QUESTION

- The problem can be broad, but it must be specific enough to convince others that it is worth focusing on.
- Research questions must be clearly delineated.
- The research questions must sometimes be delineated with sub questions.
- The scope of the research question(s) needs to be manageable within the time frame and context of the study.

PURPOSE OF THE QUALITATIVE STUDY

- Discovery?
- Description?
- Conceptualization (theory building)?
- Sensitization?
- Emancipation?
- Other?

LITERATURE REVIEW

- The literature review should be selective and persuasive, building a case for what is known or believed, what is missing, and how the study fits in.
- The literature is used to demonstrate openness to the complexity of the phenomenon, rather than funneling toward an a priori conceptualization.

METHODS—CHALLENGES HERE

- Quantitative designs are often more familiar to reviewers.
- Qualitative researchers have a different language.

METHODS SECTION

- Orientation to the method:
  - Description of the particular method that will be used and its creators/interpreters
  - Rationale for qualitative research generally and for the specific method to be used

QUALITATIVE STUDIES ARE VALUABLE FOR RESEARCH

- It delves deeply into complexities and processes.
- It focuses on little-known phenomena or innovative systems.

- It explores informal and unstructured processes in organizations.
- It seeks to explore where and why policy and local knowledge and practice are at odds.
- It is based on real, as opposed to stated, organizational goals.
- It cannot be done experimentally for practical or ethical reasons.
- It requires identification of relevant variables (Marshall & Rossman, 1999).

SAMPLE

- Purposive or theoretical sampling
  - The purpose of the sampling
  - Characteristics of potential types of persons, events, or processes to be sampled
  - Methods of making decisions about sampling
- Sample size
  - Estimates provided based on previous experience, pilot work, etc.
- Access and recruitment

DATA COLLECTION AND ANALYSIS

- Types: Individual interviews, participant observation, focus groups, personal and public documents, Internet-based data, videos, and so on, all of which vary with different traditions.
- Analysis methods vary depending on the qualitative approach.
- Add DETAILS and MORE DETAILS about how data will be gathered and processed (procedures should be made public).

QUESTIONS FOR DATA MANAGEMENT AND ANALYSIS

- How will data be kept organized and retrievable?
- How will data be "broken up" to see something new?
- How will the researchers engage in reflexivity (e.g., be self-analytical)?
- How will the reader be convinced that the researcher is sufficiently knowledgeable about qualitative analysis and has the necessary skills?

TRUSTWORTHINESS (SOUNDNESS OF THE RESEARCH)

- Should be reflected throughout the proposal
- Should be addressed specifically, with the relevant criteria for the qualitative approach used
- Should provide examples of the strategies used:
  - Triangulation
  - Prolonged contact with informants, including continuous validation of data
  - Continuous checking for representativeness of data and fit between coding categories and data
  - Use of expert consultants

EXAMPLES OF STRATEGIES FOR LIMITING BIAS IN INTERPRETATIONS

- Planning to search for negative cases
- Describing how analysis will include a purposeful examination of alternative explanations
- Using members of the research team to critically question the analysis
- Planning to conduct an audit of data collection and analytic strategies

OTHER COMPONENTS

- Ethical considerations
  - Consent forms
  - Dealing with sensitive issues
- Dissemination and knowledge translation
- Timeline
- Budget justification

LAST BITS OF ADVICE

- Seek assistance and pre-review from others with experience in grant writing (plan time for rewriting).
- Highlight match between your proposal and purpose of competition.
- Follow the rules of the competition.
- Write for a multidisciplinary audience.

REFERENCES

Marshall, C., & Rossman, G. B. (1999). *Designing qualitative research*. Thousand Oaks, CA: Sage.

Morse, J. M. (1994). Designing funded qualitative research. In N. Denzin & Y. Lincoln (Eds.), *Handbook of qualitative research* (pp. 220–235). Thousand Oaks, CA: Sage.

Silverman, D. (2000). *Doing qualitative research*. Thousand Oaks, CA: Sage.

OUTLINE FOR A RESEARCH PROPOSAL

Mary de Chesnay

*T*he following guidelines are meant as a general set of suggestions that supplement the instructions for the student's program. In all cases where there is conflicting advice, the student should be guided by the dissertation chair's instructions. The outlined plan includes five chapters: the first three constitute the proposal and the remaining two the results and conclusions, but the number may vary depending on the nature of the topic or the style of the committee chair (e.g., I do not favor repeating the research questions at the beginning of every chapter, but some faculty do. I like to use this outline but some faculty prefer a different order. Some studies lend themselves to four instead of five chapters.).

Chapter I: Overview of the Study (or Preview of Coming Attractions) is a few pages that tell the reader:

- What he or she is going to investigate (purpose or statement of the problem and research questions or hypotheses).
- What theoretical support the idea has (conceptual framework or theoretical support). In qualitative research, this section may include only a rationale for conducting the study, with the conceptual framework or typology emerging from the data.
- What assumptions underlie the problem.
- What definitions of terms are important to state (typically, these definitions in quantitative research are called *operational definitions* because they describe how one will know the item when one sees it. An operational definition usually starts with the phrase: "a score of ... or above on the [name of instrument]"). One may also want to include a conceptual definition, which is the usual meaning of the concept of interest or a definition according to a specific author. In contrast, qualitative research usually does not include measurements, so operational definitions are not appropriate, but conceptual definitions may be important to state.

- What limitations to the design are expected (not delimitations, which are intentional decisions about how to narrow the scope of one's population or focus).
- What the importance of the study (significance) is to the discipline.

Chapter II: The Review of Research Literature (or Why You Are Not Reinventing the Wheel)

For Quantitative Research:

Organize this chapter according to the concepts in the conceptual framework in Chapter I and describe the literature review thoroughly first, followed by the state of the art of the literature and how the study fills the gaps in the existing literature. Do not include non research literature in this section—place it in Chapter I as introductory material if the citation is necessary to the description.

- Concept 1: a brief description of each study reviewed that supports concept 1 with appropriate transitional statements between paragraphs
- Concept 2: a brief description of each study reviewed that supports concept 2 with appropriate transitional statements between paragraphs
- Concept 3: a brief description of each study reviewed that supports concept 3 with appropriate transitional statements between paragraphs
- And so on, for as many concepts as there are in the conceptual framework (I advise limiting the number of concepts for a master's degree thesis owing to time and cost constraints)
- Areas of agreement in the literature—a paragraph, or two, that summarizes the main points on which authors agree
- Areas of disagreement—where the main issues on which authors disagree are summarized
- State of the art on the topic—a few paragraphs in which the areas where the literature is strong and where the gaps are, are clearly articulated
- A brief statement of how the study fills the gaps or why the study needs to be conducted to replicate what someone else has done

For Qualitative Research:

The literature review is usually conducted after the results are analyzed and the emergent concepts are known. The literature may then be placed in Chapter II of the proposal as shown earlier or incorporated into the results and discussion.

Chapter III: Methodology (or Exactly What You Are Going to Do Anyway)

- Design (name the design—e.g., ethnographic, experimental, survey, cross-sectional, phenomenological, grounded theory, etc.).
- Sample—describe the number of people who will serve as the sample and the sampling method: Where and how will the sample be recruited? Provide the rationale for sample selection and methods. Include the institutional review board (IRB) statement and say how the rights of subjects (Ss) will be protected, including how informed consent will be obtained and the data coded and stored.
- Setting—where will data collection take place? In quantitative research, this might be a laboratory or, if a questionnaire, a home. If qualitative, there are special considerations of privacy and comfortable surroundings for the interviews.
- Instruments and data analysis—how will the variables of interest be measured and how will sense be made of the data, if quantitative, and if qualitative, how will the data be coded and interpreted—that is, for both, this involves how the data will be analyzed.
- Validity and reliability—how will it be known if the data are good (in qualitative research, these terms are "accuracy" and "replicability").
- Procedures for data collection and analysis: a 1-2-3 step-by-step plan for what will be done.
- Timeline—a chart that lists the plan month by month—use Month 1, 2, 3 instead of January, February, March.

The above three-chapter plan constitutes an acceptable proposal for a research project. The following is an outline for the final two chapters.

Chapter IV: Results (What I Discovered)

- Some researchers like to describe the sample in this section as a way to lead off talking about the findings.
- In the order of each hypothesis or research question, describe the data that addressed that question. Use raw data only; do not conclude anything about the data and make no interpretations.

Chapter V: Discussion (or How I Can Make Sense of All This)

- Conclusions—a concise statement of the answer to each research question or hypothesis. Some people like to interpret here—that is, to say how confident they can be about each conclusion.

- Implications—how each conclusion can be used to help address the needs of vulnerable populations or nursing practice, education, or administration.
- Recommendations for further research—that is, what will be done for an encore?

INDEX

Made in the USA
Monee, IL
27 January 2020